T0224689

# WOMEN'S JOURNEYS TO POSTTRAUMATIC GROWTH

This accessible book draws on research around women's experiences to illustrate and explore the concept of posttraumatic growth, emphasizing practice implications for healthcare professionals and strategies for fostering posttraumatic growth.

Including the voices of women, in their own words, *Women's Journeys to Posttraumatic Growth* explains the differences between posttraumatic stress disorder and posttraumatic growth and presents the theoretical framework of posttraumatic growth. It synthesizes relevant international research and introduces data from four new qualitative research studies on posttraumatic growth in women who have experienced the death of a spouse or longtime partner, death of a child, a close brush with death, and intimate partner abuse. The book develops clinical and nursing practice implications for healthcare professionals and explores current self-help and professional therapeutic strategies to foster posttraumatic growth.

*Women's Journeys to Posttraumatic Growth* is an invaluable guide for health and social care practitioners, as well as students and researchers with an interest in trauma, abuse, bereavement and loss, and women's healthcare.

**Mary Ellen Doherty** is professor of nursing at Western Connecticut State University, USA. Most of her career has been spent in clinical practice as a certified nurse midwife; she has delivered over 2,000 babies in her midwifery career. She was founder and president of Concord Midwifery Associates with delivery privileges at Emerson Hospital in Concord, Massachusetts. She is an active researcher on women's health topics and midwifery care. Dr. Doherty was the 2012 recipient of the Norton Mezvinsky Award for Excellence in Research. She is a fellow of the American College of Nurse-Midwives.

**Elizabeth Scannell-Desch** is retired associate dean at Rutgers University, School of Nursing, Camden, USA. She holds the tenured rank of professor. Elizabeth retired from the U.S. Air Force (Nurse Corps) in 1997, after serving on active duty for 25 years. Dr. Scannell-Desch attained the rank of colonel, and her last assignment was at the Pentagon. Elizabeth was a visiting professor at the University of Medicine and Pharmacy, Cluj-Napoka, Romania. Her program of research has focused on women's health issues and military nursing. She is a fellow of the American Academy of Nursing.

'An empathetic exploration of women's traumas and how those experiencing them travel to Posttraumatic Growth. The authors explore the tumultuous emotions stirred up by the death of a loved one, domestic abuse, serious accidents, illnesses, and the broad fluctuations between hope and despair. Insightful, practical, compassionate, and a must-read!'

**Sharon R. Rainer, Ph.D., APRN, FNP-BC, ANP-BC, ENP-C**,
*Program Director, Emergency Nurse Practitioner Post-Graduate Program,*
*Thomas Jefferson University College of Nursing, USA*

'*Women's Journeys to Posttraumatic Growth* is compassionately infused with true stories of life traumas encountered by ordinary women. Drs. Doherty and Scannell-Desch draw on their research and clinical experience to provide the reader with a riveting account of women's struggles, setbacks, and gradual navigation to Posttraumatic Growth.'

**Iris J. Turkenkopf, Ph.D.**, *Professor & Vice President for Academic Affairs (retired), Mount Saint Mary College, USA*

# WOMEN'S JOURNEYS TO POSTTRAUMATIC GROWTH

A Guide for the Helping Professions and Women Who Have Experienced Trauma

*Mary Ellen Doherty and Elizabeth Scannell-Desch*

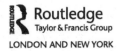
Routledge
Taylor & Francis Group

LONDON AND NEW YORK

Designed cover image: © Getty Images

First published 2024

by Routledge
4 Park Square, Milton Park, Abingdon, Oxon OX14 4RN

and by Routledge
605 Third Avenue, New York, NY 10158

*Routledge is an imprint of the Taylor & Francis Group, an informa business*

© 2024 Mary Ellen Doherty and Elizabeth Scannell-Desch

The right of Mary Ellen Doherty and Elizabeth Scannell-Desch to be identified as authors of this work has been asserted in accordance with sections 77 and 78 of the Copyright, Designs and Patents Act 1988.

All rights reserved. No part of this book may be reprinted or reproduced or utilised in any form or by any electronic, mechanical, or other means, now known or hereafter invented, including photocopying and recording, or in any information storage or retrieval system, without permission in writing from the publishers.

*Trademark notice*: Product or corporate names may be trademarks or registered trademarks, and are used only for identification and explanation without intent to infringe.

*British Library Cataloguing-in-Publication Data*
A catalogue record for this book is available from the British Library

ISBN: 978-1-032-59868-0 (hbk)
ISBN: 978-1-032-59866-6 (pbk)
ISBN: 978-1-003-45665-0 (ebk)

DOI: 10.4324/9781003456650

Typeset in Optima
by SPi Technologies India Pvt Ltd (Straive)

*This book is personally dedicated to Maeve Marie and Sophia Angela, two little girls, who will grow up to change the world and make it a better place.*

*This book is professionally dedicated to Sister Leona DeBoer, OP, RN, Ph.D., professor, mentor, and role model in our nursing careers, who guided us on the path toward clinical practice, education, and research many years ago.*

*It is also dedicated to the brave women who have shared their stories with us to give voice to their traumatic experiences. Their words serve to educate all of us about trauma and its aftermath and the possibility of posttraumatic growth.*

# CONTENTS

# FOREWORD

It has been my privilege to know both authors, **Mary Ellen Doherty** and **Elizabeth Scannell-Desch**, not only as educators, clinicians, and researchers but as true humanitarians. Through their numerous journal publications and three books, they have increased society's awareness of how the human spirit can overcome various traumatic experiences and then progress through life in a positive manner. This book, *Women's Journeys to Posttraumatic Growth: A Guide for the Helping Professions and Women Who Have Experienced Trauma*, adds to the awareness, as it explores the traumatic experiences of women and their subsequent reestablishment of their lives.

The ability of these authors to compassionately elicit the detail and reflection from each woman in telling their traumatic experiential story is what distinguishes this book and allows the reader to gain increased insight into the tools used to navigate recovery. This reader came away with increased knowledge of responses to trauma and decisions about paths to recovery, which is exceedingly helpful not only to anyone engaged in a helping profession but to those who have experienced similar traumatic life circumstances.

Trauma is something everyone is aware of and usually fears due to the perceived loss of control it brings. As I read through the chapters of this book, I was taken on a journey through the depths of sadness, loss, fear, and despair but came away enlightened by the fortitude, determination, and optimism these women found within themselves to travel forward despite grappling with tragic life circumstances.

Thank you to the authors and women who shared their experiences in this book. Many of these stories I will never forget. As a mental health clinician, I have learned a great deal about the possibility of posttraumatic growth through reading this book. I found the references used in each chapter to be extremely comprehensive, and the bibliography at the end of chapters was a huge plus.

This book serves as a guide for all clinicians and anyone dealing with a traumatic life experience. The narratives demonstrate trauma and adversity, as well as the strength of the human spirit, and how victimization can be replaced with increased posttraumatic growth.

**Christine M. Berté, EdD, APRN, FNP-BC, CNE**

# PREFACE

This book was born from four qualitative research studies examining the concept of *posttraumatic growth* (PTG) in four distinct groups of women. PTG is a lesser-known but related concept to *posttraumatic stress disorder* (PTSD). PTG was defined in the 1990s by two psychology professors, Drs. Richard Tedeschi and Lawrence Calhoun, at the University of North Carolina in Charlotte. They described PTG as "the positive personal transformations that can occur in the aftermath of trauma" (Tedeschi & Calhoun, 1995 1996, 2004). PTSD can be a chronic and psychological, social, and spiritual condition that affects a wide variety of people, their families, and society. It is a response that can be linked to traumatic experiences such as accidents, war, natural disasters, violent assaults, and domestic abuse.

Before our research for this book, we initially studied 9/11 widows who were pregnant at the time of the tragedy and who went on to have their babies without the presence of their deceased partners. Then, we studied the experiences of U.S. military nurses who served in the war-torn countries of Iraq and Afghanistan. Later, we studied their reintegration experiences after returning home from war. The stories of the nurses were not always about the psychological and physical trauma that stems from war. Their stories sometimes told of positive changes they made in their lives after dealing with adversity. Many nurses found meaning and purpose in their lives. Some discovered that they needed a clinical change of scenery which offered new possibilities.

Our two previous books, *Nurses in War: Voices from Iraq and Afghanistan* (Scannell-Desch & Doherty, 2012) and *Nurses After War: The Reintegration Experience of Nurses Returning from Iraq and Afghanistan* (Doherty & Scannell-Desch, 2016) gave testimony to the trauma experienced during and after these two wars. Yet, some stories exemplified satisfaction, fulfillment, and understanding that transformed the nurses' lives. These stories (Scannell-Desch & Doherty, 2012; Doherty & Scannell-Desch, 2016) illustrated the concept of PTG. While an exploration of PTG was not the intent of this research, elements of it were evident in the stories of the nurses during their combat exposure and their reintegration. Therefore, our interest in PTG was sparked as a result of our previous research. We knew that we wanted to explore and describe PTG in greater detail with subsequent research.

The current book, *Women's Journeys to Posttraumatic Growth: A Guide for the Helping Professions and Women Who Have Experienced Trauma*, is based on four qualitative research studies of women who have faced adversity. Each study focused on a distinct group of women who had experienced the same type of traumatic experience. These groups were women who have experienced the loss of a spouse/partner, the loss of a child, a close brush with death, and domestic abuse. We chose these four groups of women based on our nursing experience as clinicians, professors, and researchers.

The purpose of this book is to inform and educate the reader about the possibility of PTG. While the book was written for a target group, nurses and other healthcare providers, it is hoped that the narratives and commentary contained in this book will be helpful and meaningful not only to those involved in healthcare settings but to all readers. No one's life is without challenges, and we consider every person on the planet to be individual and unique.

Thus, everyone is different and varies in their life experiences and belief system. The book will take the reader on an interesting and enlightening journey exploring PTG through the real-life stories of women as they dissected and detailed their traumatic experiences through the lens of PTG. The researchers merely asked the questions, and usually this was all that was needed to open the floodgates of emotions and memories for each study participant. Their stories touched on a myriad of experiences, challenges, emotions, and pain but also highlighted personal triumphs, support, strength, and love. The first study was comprised of 14 women who had lost their husbands to death. None of the deaths had been within five years of the interviews. This was a decision made by the researchers to allow some healing to take place and a chance for the participants to gain some perspective regarding their loss. Purposive sampling was employed using the researchers' nursing network of colleagues from academic institutions, hospital affiliations, and professional nursing organizations. The study began with in-person interviews but had to be changed to telephone interviews because of Covid-19 pandemic restrictions. Five themes merged from data analysis: (1) anticipated loss, (2) unanticipated loss, (3) a new depth of compassion and empathy, (4) my strength grew over time, and (5) my view of myself changed.

In the second study, the 13 participants included 11 mothers and two grandmothers. The researchers made an exception for the grandmothers because both women wanted to participate in the study, having been present when their newborn granddaughters died. The loss was "up close and personal," and both women thought they could contribute to the narratives regarding the profound loss of a child. All interviews for this study were conducted telephonically because of pandemic restrictions. Again, the researchers used their nursing network to recruit participants for the study. Seven themes emerged from data analysis: (1) when my child died, I lost part of myself; (2) anticipated loss versus unanticipated loss; (3) picking up the pieces of my life; (4) support, kindness, and compassion helped; (5) moving on while still broken; (6) never forgotten, always in my heart; and (7) holding my loved ones close.

The third study was comprised of 12 women who had experienced a close brush with death by their estimation. Experiences included cardiac events, cancer, serious infections and illnesses, a violent assault, a near-drowning, a motor vehicle accident, and a plane crash. Three interviews were in-person, and the remainder were via telephone. Both geographic distance and pandemic restrictions affected how the interview was conducted. The researchers used their nursing network of colleagues from academic institutions, clinical affiliations, public health facilities, and professional nursing organizations to identify potential participants. The final sample was 12 women. Seven themes emerged from data analysis. They included (1) when trauma happens; (2) the will to survive; (3) support: I'm not alone; (4) a second chance at life; (5) I'm stronger than I thought I was; (6) putting the pieces of my life back together; and (7) near-death experiences: some women had them.

In the fourth study, 14 women reported emotional and/or physical abuse by their male partners. Interview data were analyzed by qualitative content analysis. Many women considered verbal abuse, which consisted of threats, name-calling, gaslighting, isolation, and various forms of control, to be more significant and hurtful than physical abuse. Of the 14 participants, 13 women had left their abuser. The one remaining woman, who was elderly, stayed married to her abusive husband. This woman had support from her eight adult children and numerous friends and relatives. She had made a life for herself despite her husband's long-standing bad behavior. Five themes were identified: (1) acknowledging the abusive relationship; (2) fear of him: threats, control, pain, and isolation; (3) accepting support: grabbing the life preserver; (4) rediscovering myself: digging deep; and (5) appreciating life and helping others.

Data-generating open-ended questions guided the interview process in all four studies. Follow-up questions were asked to clarify words, thoughts, feelings, and meanings of what was expressed, and to gain a greater understanding of the content. Reflective questions were asked, and suggestive or leading questions were avoided.

The four study proposals were approved by institutional review boards where the researchers were employed. Before interviews were scheduled, potential participants were mailed a typed information sheet outlining the basic tenets of the study as well as an informed consent form. The researchers did not schedule any interviews until a signed consent form was received. Then, one of the researchers contacted the participants by telephone to see if they had any questions about the study and to schedule an interview. Participants were given the option of an in-person or telephone interview depending on geographic distance, personal schedule, and Covid-19 pandemic restrictions. Participation was voluntary and could be withdrawn at any time. Participants were informed of the immediate availability of a mental health nurse practitioner if needed, because of the possibility that a participant could become upset while describing their memories of trauma. Procedures for data collection, analysis, storage, and use were explained. All interviews were audio-recorded for the accuracy of data and transcribed verbatim by the researchers. Data collection for each study took approximately one year with occasional pauses because of Covid-19 pandemic restrictions, schedule changes, and participant availability. In addition, data collection and analysis were dictated by the achievement of data saturation.

Data analysis for the four studies used procedures of qualitative content analysis (Polit & Beck, 2017; Elo & Kyngas, 2008; Schreier, 2012). Audio-taped interviews were listened to several times by both researchers to gain familiarity with the content, feeling, and tone. Then, the verbatim transcriptions were reviewed, and significant statements were highlighted and categorized into theme clusters. Each final theme was indicative of the words and sentiments of the majority of the participants in each study. Although all experiences and interview content were valued, it was not possible to include every word that was said in an interview in this book. Statements that best capture the themes were included in this book.

Extraneous, off-topic, and inconsequential words or ideas were omitted for the sake of clarity and when the researchers deemed that the conversation was not necessary, meaning that it did not add to the description. The reader of this book will be introduced to 14 widows who share their stories of loss and who mention elements of PTG in their narratives. The widowhood literature is replete with examples illustrating the significant impact of the loss of a spouse or long-term partner. Widowhood can challenge a woman's psychological, physical, social, spiritual, and economic well-being. Women dealing with loss are faced with significant stressors which place them at risk for a variety of health problems. The reader will also obtain a lens into the heartbreaking experience of losing a child to death. Eleven mothers and two grandmothers provided a window into this devastating experience. They described the circumstances, emotions, pain, and aftermath of suffering. Bereaved mothers and grandmothers were forced to deal with the core questions of human existence. These women had to face the disruption of what is perceived to be the natural course of life, with children outliving their parents and grandparents. The impact of losing a child or grandchild can persist for many years. The third research study gives the reader a firsthand account of what it is like to stare death in the face. Some participants expressed feelings that they would not recover and were surprised that they survived. Others talked about their strong will to live, and the support they received from nurses and other healthcare providers as well as their family, friends, and co-workers. Many survivors acknowledged spirituality, religion, and their belief in God as a source of comfort. Thankfulness and gratitude were mentioned repeatedly in the women's stories. Several women told of their newfound desire to help others experiencing ill health and injuries.

The fourth study focused on 14 women who experienced domestic abuse, whether it be emotional, physical, or both. This study specifically addresses a gap in the abuse literature about PTG. The use of control was a dominant factor and a significant component in the women's stories. Some women saw a pivotal change in their husband's behavior after marriage. Others felt like prisoners or indentured servants in their own homes. Gaslighting was another commonplace tactic for exerting power, control, and isolation. Every participant in this study, except for one elderly woman, chose to leave their abuser. The PTG framework was useful in examining women's experiences. Pseudonyms were used in the four research studies to maintain anonymity for the research participants. All participants signed informed consent documents and agreed to have their interviews audio-recorded and transcribed verbatim. They were aware that research studies are often presented in a scholarly forum at professional conferences sponsored by a nursing organization or academic institution. In addition, they also knew that research studies are often published in academic and professional journals. Any statement that is enclosed in quotation marks was recorded in a formal interview and represents that person's recollection of events.

We are grateful to the strong and resourceful women who chose to share their stories with us in the name of nursing science and knowledge development. They hoped that other women would benefit from their words, sentiments, and experiences. We acknowledge and respect their courage, honesty, and integrity for agreeing to participate in our research.

## References

Doherty, M. E., & Scannell-Desch, E. A. (2016). *Nurses after war: The reintegration experience of nurses returning from Iraq and Afghanistan*, Springer.

Elo, A., & Kyngas, H. (2008). The qualitative content analysis process. *Journal of Advanced Nursing* 62(1), 107–115.

Polit, D. F., & Beck, C. T. (2017). *Nursing research: Principles and methods*. Lippincott, Williams, and Wilkins.

Scannell-Desch, E. A., & Doherty, M. E. (2012). *Nurses in war: Voices from Iraq and Afghanistan*, Springer.

Schreier, M. (2012). *Qualitative content analysis in practice*. Sage.

Tedeschi, R., & Calhoun, L. (1995). *Trauma and transformation: Growth in the aftermath of suffering*. Sage.

Tedeschi, R., & Calhoun, L. (1996). The posttraumatic growth inventory: Measuring the positive legacy of trauma. *Journal of Traumatic Stress*, *9*(3), 455–472.

Tedeschi, R., & Calhoun, L. (2004). Posttraumatic growth: Conceptual foundations and empirical evidence. *Psychological Inquiry*, *15*, 1–18.

# ACKNOWLEDGEMENTS

This book could not have been written without the support of family, friends, and nursing colleagues. We wish to thank Len, Chris, Meaghan, Jake, Maxwell, and Maggie for their support, kindness, and love.

# ABBREVIATIONS

| | |
|---|---|
| ADD | Attention deficit disorder |
| BDI | Beck Depression Inventory |
| CBT | Cognitive behavioral therapy |
| C-Diff | Clostridium deficile |
| Covid-19 | Coronavirus 2019 |
| CPT | Cognitive processing therapy |
| D&C | Dilation and curettage |
| EMDR | Eye movement desensitization and reprocessing |
| EMT | Emergency medical technician |
| IES-R | Impact Event Scale-Revised |
| IRB | Institutional review board |
| MBSR | Mindfulness-based stress reduction program |
| MI | Myocardial infarction |
| MRSA | Methicillin-resistant Staphylococcus aureus |
| NDEs | Near-death experiences |
| NICU | Neonatal Intensive Care Unit |
| PCL-5 | Posttraumatic stress checklist |
| PTG | Posttraumatic growth |
| PTSD | Post-traumatic stress disorder |
| PET | Prolonged exposure Therapy |
| RSV | Respiratory syncytial virus |
| TPN | Total parenteral nutrition |
| SSRIs | Selective serotonin reuptake inhibitors |
| TEE | Transesophageal endoscopy |

# 1

# BEFORE POSTTRAUMATIC GROWTH CAME POSTTRAUMATIC STRESS

It is important to recognize that posttraumatic growth (PTG) can eventually occur in the years following a traumatic event and subsequent posttraumatic stress. Posttraumatic stress disorder (PTSD) is a topic and mental health disorder that has usually been associated in the media as a disorder in veterans who have experienced combat-related stresses. It became an official mental health diagnosis in 1980 after centuries of notable descriptions of a variety of symptoms by medical professionals during and after many wars around the globe. Research about soldiers returning from war was a significant piece of the creation of the PTSD diagnosis. So, the history of what is now known as PTSD often traces its roots to a history of veteran experiences in war (Weisaeth, 2014).

Descriptions of psychological symptoms following military trauma date back to ancient times. The American Civil War (1861–1865) and the Franco-Prussian War (1870–1871) indicate the start of formal medical efforts to address the difficulties of soldiers exposed to combat. Before US military medical efforts to describe PTSD and its symptoms, Austrian physicians in the late 1700s wrote about "nostalgia" among soldiers. Among those who were exposed to battlefield trauma, some reported missing home, sadness, sleep problems, and anxiety. This description of PTSD-like symptoms was a model of psychological injury that existed in the US Civil War. US military physicians studied Civil War soldiers who demonstrated a rapid heartbeat, anxiety, jumpiness, and difficulty breathing. They called this cluster of symptoms "soldier's heart" and described these symptoms as over-stimulation of the heart's nervous system. These soldiers were usually returned to the battlefield after receiving drugs to control their symptoms (Wilson, 1994).

During and after World War I, military physicians coined the term "shellshock" because of the cluster of symptoms observed in soldiers such as shaking, panic attacks, nightmares, anxiety, sleep disorders, and even disorientation that were seen as a reaction to the explosion of artillery shells in the trenches in France. Shellshock was first thought to be the result of hidden damage to the brain caused by the impact of exploding artillery. Medical thinking changed when more soldiers who had not been near explosions had similar symptoms. "War neurosis" was also a label given to this cluster of symptoms during World War I. During World War I, treatment for this cluster of symptoms varied.

DOI: 10.4324/9781003456650-1

Soldiers often received only a few days of rest before returning to the war zone. For those with severe or chronic symptoms, treatments focused on activities of daily living such as bathing, eating, dressing, and grooming appropriately to increase functioning in expectation of returning these veterans to productive civilian lives (Figley & Boscarino, 2012).

In World War II, the shellshock diagnosis was replaced by "combat stress reaction," also known as "battle fatigue." With the long operational campaigns of World War II, troops became battle weary and exhausted. Approximately half of World War II military medical discharges were the result of combat fatigue because many soldiers who were diagnosed with this symptom cluster were deemed unfit to return to the war zone. The military medical establishment tried to treat those with physical injuries as well as combat fatigue casualties without delay to return those with combat fatigue symptomatology to the war zone after a reasonable rest period and make sure sufferers expected complete recovery so that they could return to combat after rest. The benefits of military unit cohesive relationships and support became a focus of both preventing stress and promoting recovery (US Department of Veteran Affairs, 2017).

The American Psychological Association (APA) added PTSD to the *Diagnostic and Statistical Manual of Mental Disorders–III* (DSM-III; American Psychological Association, 1980) which stemmed from research involving returning Vietnam War veterans, Holocaust survivors, rape and sexual trauma victims, victims of torture, and those who survived other natural and man-made disasters such as earthquakes, hurricanes, explosions, aircraft crashes, and major fires and shipwrecks. The DSM-III criteria for PTSD were revised in DSM-III-R (American Psychological Association, 1987), DSM-IV (American Psychological Association, 1994), DSM-IV-TR (American Psychological Association, 2000), and DSM-V (American Psychological Association, 2013) to reflect continuing research surrounding this disorder. A significant finding, which was not well-defined at first, is that PTSD is relatively commonplace. Recent data shows about 4 out of every 100 American men (or 4%) and 10 out of every 100 American women (or 10%) will be diagnosed with PTSD at some time in their life (US Department of Veteran Affairs, 2017; Weathers et al., 2013).

Since the publishing of DSM-III, PTSD is no longer considered an anxiety disorder. A new diagnostic category was added, labeled, "Trauma-and Stressor-Related Disorders."

PTSD includes four types of symptom categories:

- Reliving the trauma—flashbacks, hallucinations, nightmares of the traumatic event
- Avoiding the trauma—avoiding people, places, things, or memories that remind you of the traumatic event
- Excessive arousal of the trauma—increased alertness (hyper-alertness), anger, fits of rage, irritability, or difficulty sleeping or concentrating
- Intrusive negative distressing thoughts or feelings, such as guilt
- Flat affect.

*(Geier et al., 2019)*

Most people experience some of these symptoms after a traumatic event, so PTSD is not diagnosed unless all four types of symptoms last for at least a month and cause significant distress or problems with day-to-day activities and functioning (Tanielian, 2008).

In terms of this book, we provided information about PTSD because many women who lose a spouse, bury a child, have a near-death experience, or suffer from intimate partner abuse are likely to have either been diagnosed with PTSD or have undiagnosed PTSD. Other psychiatric diagnoses such as depression, generalized anxiety disorder, and suicidal ideation may also accompany the diagnosis of PTSD. Mental health therapies currently used in the treatment of PTSD include cognitive processing therapy (CPT), prolonged exposure therapy (PET), and eye movement desensitization and reprocessing (EMDR) (Rothbaum et al., 2005). In addition, medications such as selective serotonin reuptake inhibitors (SSRIs) and antidepressants are sometimes prescribed for clients suffering from PTSD (Ehlers et al., 2013; Lee et al., 2016). More information on treatment modalities is covered in Chapter 7.

## References

American Psychological Association. (1980). *Diagnostic and statistical manual of mental disorders* (3rd ed.). APA.

American Psychological Association. (1987). *Diagnostic and statistical manual of mental disorders* (3rd ed., revised). APA.

American Psychological Association. (1994). *Diagnostic and statistical manual of mental disorders* (4th ed.). APA.

American Psychological Association. (2000). *Diagnostic and statistical manual of mental disorders* (4th ed., TR). APA.

American Psychological Association. (2013). *Diagnostic and statistical manual of mental disorders* (5th ed.). APA.

Ehlers, A., Grey, N., & Wild, J. (2013). Implementation of cognitive therapy for PTSD in routine clinical care: Effectiveness and moderators of outcome in a consecutive sample. *Behavioral Research Therapy, 51*(11), 742–752.

Figley, C. R., & Boscarino, J. A. (2012). The traumatology of life. *Journal of Nervous and Mental Disorders, 200*(12), 1113–1120. https://doi.org/10.1097/NMD.0b013e318275d559

Geier, T. J., Hunt, J. C., Nelson, L. D., Brasel, K. J., & deRoon-Cassini, T.A. (2019). Detecting PTSD in a traumatically injured population: The diagnostic utility of the PTSD checklist for DSM-5. *Depression and Anxiety, 36*(2), 170–178.

Lee, D. J., Schnitzlein, C. W., Wolf, J. P., Vythilingam, M., Rasmusson, A. M., & Hoge, C. W. (2016). Psychotherapy versus pharmacotherapy for posttraumatic stress disorder: Systemic review and meta-analyses to determine first-line treatments. *Depression and Anxiety, 33*(9), 792–806.

Rothbaum, B. O., Astin, M. C., & Marsteller, F. (2005). Prolonged exposure versus eye movement desensitization and reprocessing (EMDR) for PTSD rape victims. *Journal of Trauma and Stress, 18*(6), 607–616.

Tanielian, T. (2008). *Invisible wounds of war: Psychological and cognitive injuries, their consequences, and services to assist recovery.* RAND Corporation.

US Department of Veteran Affairs, Department of Defense. (2017). *VA/DOD clinical practice guideline for the management of posttraumatic stress disorder and acute stress disorder.* The Management of Posttraumatic Stress Disorder Work Group, 1–200.

Weathers, F, Litz, B, Keane, T, Palmieri, P, Marx, B, & Schnurr, P (2013). *The PTSD checklist for DSM-5 (PCL-5). Scale available from the National Center for PTSD.* National Center for PTSD.

Weisaeth, L. (2014). The history of psychic trauma. In M. J. Friedman, T. M. Keane, & P. A. Resick (Eds.), *Handbook of PTSD: Science and practice* (pp. 38–59). Guilford Press.

Wilson, J. P. (1994). The historical evolution of PTSD diagnostic criteria. *Journal of Traumatic Stress, 7*(4), 681–698. https://doi.org/10.1007/02103015f/BF

# 2

# A CONCEPTUAL FRAMEWORK AND MODEL FOR POSTTRAUMATIC GROWTH

Conceptual frameworks are used in research studies to provide a focus. They describe a perspective in which key factors or elements such as constructs or variables link to relationships (Roberts & Hyatt, 2019). These frameworks set boundaries and provide a foundation for the construction of a research study. The use of a framework helps to ground the study within the research design. Thus, the research problem or question is a fundamental building block within the study's design. The framework provides the scaffolding for the study and helps limit the scope of the study.

The term posttraumatic growth (PTG) was coined by two psychology professors, Drs. Richard Tedeschi and Lawrence Calhoun, at the University of North Carolina in Charlotte in the 1990s. They introduced the term to describe positive psychological changes occurring after a struggle from traumatic, painful, and highly challenging life circumstances (Tedeschi & Calhoun, 1995, 1996, 2004). It is important to recognize that when humans are forced to deal with adversity, the restoration of psychological functioning and well-being is certainly a possibility. While these psychologists acknowledge that traumatic events can lead to feelings of distress, extreme sadness, vulnerability, and anger, they have also seen people emerge after struggling with adverse circumstances to make positive changes in their lives.

PTG exceeds resilience, which is described as a process of managing and adapting to significant sources of stress or trauma. Resources within an individual, their life history, and their environment facilitate a capacity to "bounce back" in times of adversity. Thus, PTG is more than simply "bouncing back" to one's previous level of functioning. With PTG, the person goes on to function at a higher level because of the lessons learned from the struggle. However, a person can experience PTG and PTSD at the same time. This is referred to as one of the paradoxes of PTG, meaning that from loss there can be gain. It is not by any means an either/or situation; it is complex and multifaceted because of the nature of the trauma and the coping, healing, and recovery trajectory of the person. We were able to see the development of PTG in some of the women who participated in the research studies discussed in this book. Examples include women who were able to help others after losing a child, women who chose to volunteer at safe houses and shelters after surviving domestic abuse themselves, and women who became involved in humanitarian

DOI: 10.4324/9781003456650-2

organizations after dealing with their trauma. Many women expressed a desire to give back, move forward, and live a life full of gratitude and strength with an open mind and firm purpose.

Growth after adversity can be traced back to the early writings of the ancient Hebrews, Greeks, and Christians, as well as some of the teachings of Hinduism, Buddhism, and Islam (Linley, 2003; Tedeschi & Calhoun, 1995). It involves a shift in one's thought processes that can lead to transformation. Western culture has embraced the notion that traumatic experiences and the suffering they entail can lead to strength and personal growth (Tennen & Afleck, 2009). Much of the research about PTG involves participants' self-selection and self-report.

## The Posttraumatic Growth Model

Tedeschi and Calhoun (1996, 2004) identified five domains of PTG: (1) a greater appreciation of life, (2) improved relationships with others, (3) increased personal strength, (4) openness to new possibilities, and (5) spiritual growth. A greater appreciation of life involves a shift in one's priorities and taking time to appreciate things that might have gone unnoticed before or simply taken for granted. This usually causes a person to redefine what is important to them and to also take stock of their life lived so far. Improved relationships with others may involve holding loved ones close, appreciating one's support system, and having a renewed sense of caring for humankind. It may also include developing an increased sense of compassion and empathy. Increased personal strength may be experienced as independence, confidence, emotional balance, and self-control, illustrated by effective coping strategies and greater adaptation.

Openness to new possibilities relates to one's ability to venture outside of their comfort zone. This may involve engaging in new activities, meeting new people, making a career change, or choosing to follow one's passion rather than staying with the status quo. Spiritual growth may cause one to examine their belief system and seek meaning in life (Tedeschi & Calhoun, 1996, 2004). Some people may choose to revisit their former religion or seek new meaning in nature or the universe.

## What Does the Research Tell Us?

PTG has been studied in various groups of trauma survivors, such as cancer survivors (Soo & Sherwin, 2015), amputees (Benetato, 2011), traumatic childbirth survivors (Sawyer et al., 2012), physically abused children (Farnia et al., 2017), adult survivors of interpersonal violence (Elderton et al., 2017), disaster survivors (Holgerson et al., 2010), combat soldiers (Mark et al., 2018; Palmer et al., 2017; Tsai et al., 2016), and nurses deployed to the Iraq and Afghanistan wars (Doherty et al., 2020). However, it is important to mention that not everyone who has experienced tragedy or trauma will go on to experience PTG (Joseph & Linley, 2005; Linley & Joseph, 2005; Park, 2010). A person's emotional response to a traumatic event helps to determine the long-term outcome of that trauma. The outcome can be negatively affected by factors occurring during and after the trauma. This may increase the risk of developing PTSD (Brewin et al., 2000). Conversely, the personality characteristics of the individual and the specific circumstances of the trauma may contribute to the development of PTG (Shuwiekh et al., 2018).

According to Tedeschi and Calhoun (2004), PTG is both a process and an outcome. As a process, PTG has a beginning, a middle, and an end. The end is the outcome, such as positive changes in a person's life. It is the struggle with the trauma or tragedy that sparks the process to begin. Thus, the steps in the process can lead a person to the realization that they have developed capacities for appreciating life, relating better to others, and having personal strength.

Over time, the person starts to see themselves in a different light. Perhaps these capacities were not present before the trauma, or they were dormant or simply not recognized by the person. The traumatic experience may lead to personal strength, which can benefit the person by making them more able to face future challenges.

Posttraumatic stress is often considered a possible outcome for people who have witnessed a tragic event or directly experienced the many types of traumatic experiences one can encounter in life. While it is important to acknowledge a person's psychological response to trauma, it is also imperative to see that trauma survivors can eventually have PTG. Often, a traumatic experience can cause a person to question their belief system. They may question their purpose in life, their relationships with others, their self-worth, and the many choices and decisions they have made throughout life.

When a person is faced with extremely stressful and traumatic life-changing experiences, such as the loss of a spouse or partner, the loss of a child, experiencing a terrifyingly close brush with death, or living with the constant fear of physical violence, bullying, gaslighting, and character assassination, their assumptive world is disrupted if not destroyed. This is because the individual's world has been turned upside-down so to speak, and what they counted on as being reliable, predictable, and maybe even controllable to a certain extent is no longer the case. If the person can improve their situation by gradually rebuilding and modifying their world, they may be able to return to some semblance of order and more effective functioning. Posttraumatic growth may be the eventual outcome if the person can put the pieces of their life back together through a concerted effort and as a result of the struggle they experienced. Lessons learned are beneficial and can lead a person to a better place where they may find personal strength, a renewed appreciation for relationships with others, new opportunities for growth in many directions, a revitalized spirituality, and a reassessment of their priorities in life with a future orientation. This transformation is positive, energizing, and appreciated (Tedeschi & Calhoun, 2004). It has been noted in the literature that people with greater self-esteem tend to be more motivated and confident in their ability to work diligently to take control of their lives (Lund et al., 1993). In addition, people who embrace religion in times of crisis as a coping resource may discover enhanced meaning in life as they reconstruct their belief system in their assumptive world (Matthews & Marwit, 2006; Park et al., 1996). Both religiosity and spirituality may foster life-changing transformations of goals and priorities (Pargament & Ano, 2006) and promote a more insightful comprehension of one's purpose in life (Tedeschi & Calhoun, 2004).

It has been suggested that social support usually helps trauma victims address their challenges and consequently evokes a greater appreciation for human connection. Tedeschi and Calhoun (2004) mention that social support often allows individuals the opportunity to share their thoughts and feelings with others and obtain feedback as they face their transformed reality. In addition, they suggest that in rebuilding or reconstructing one's reality, a person engages in persistent thinking and ruminates about their radically changed reality. Eventually, if PTG has occurred, the person will come to recognize their newfound strength and will be better equipped to face future challenges (Tedeschi & Calhoun, 2004).

Tedeschi and Calhoun (2004) reported that certain personality traits may contribute to the development of PTG in a trauma victim. For example, they suggest that a person who is extraverted and open to new experiences may more easily recognize positive outcomes and emotions than someone who is reserved and introverted. An outgoing, friendly person may be more receptive to accepting support from others and they may actively seek it out. Similarly, Park et al. (1996) posit that inherently optimistic people may be more predisposed to growth after trauma because they believe that they will somehow get through the trauma or tragedy they are facing.

As researchers, we believe that it was important to conduct qualitative studies using open-ended questions to elicit honest and trustworthy responses from the participants in the four studies discussed in this book. Furthermore, we believe that individuals are more candid in their replies to open-ended questions when they have the freedom to take their time with descriptions and revelations. It is often cathartic to tell your story to an interested, patient, nonjudgmental listener.

## References

Benetato, B. (2011). Posttraumatic growth among operation enduring freedom and operation Iraqi freedom amputees. *Journal of Nursing Scholarship, 43*, 412–420.

Brewin, C. R., Andrews, B., & Valentine, J. D. (2000). Meta-analysis of risk factors for posttraumatic stress disorder in trauma-exposed adults. *Journal of Consulting and Clinical Psychology, 68*(5), 748–766.

Doherty, M. E., Scannell-Desch, E. A., & Bready, J. (2020). A positive side of deployment: Vicarious posttraumatic growth in U.S. military nurses who served in the Iraq and Afghanistan wars. *Journal of Nursing Scholarship, 52*(3), 233–241.

Elderton, A., Berry, A., & Chen, C. (2017). A systematic review of posttraumatic growth survivors of interpersonal violence. *Trauma, Violence, Abuse, 18*(2), 223–236.

Farnia, V., Tatari, F., Salami, S., Alikhani, M., & Basanj, B. (2017). Efficacy of trauma-focused cognitive behavioral therapy in facilitating emotional posttraumatic growth and emotional management among physically abused children. *Trauma Monthly, 23*, 1–6.

Holgerson, K., Boe, H., & Holen, A. (2010). Long-term perspectives on posttraumatic growth in disaster survivors. *Journal of Traumatic Stress, 23*, 413–416.

Joseph, S., & Linley, P. (2005). Positive adjustment to threatening events: An orgasmic valuing theory of growth through adversity. *Review of General Psychology, 9*(3), 262–280.

Linley. P. (2003). Positive adaptation to trauma: Wisdom as both process and outcome. *Journal of Traumatic Stress, 18*, 575–585.

Linley, P., & Joseph, S. (2005). The human capacity for growth through adversity. *American Psychologist, 60*(3), 262–264.

Lund, D. A., Caserta, M. S., & Dimond, M. F. (1993). The course of spousal bereavement in later life. In M. S. Stroebe, W. Stroebe, & R. O. Hansson (Eds.), *Handbook of bereavement: Theory, research, and intervention* (pp. 240–254). Cambridge University Press. https://doi.org/10.1017/CBO9780511664076.017

Mark, K., Stevelink, S., Choi, J., & Fear, N. (2018). Posttraumatic growth in the military: A systematic review. *Occupational and Environmental Medicine 2018, 75*(12), 904–915.

Matthews, L. T., & Marwit, S. J. (2006). Complicated grief and the trend toward cognitive-behavioral therapy. *Death Studies, 28*(9), 849–863. https://doi.org/10.1080/07481180490490924

Palmer, E., Murphy, D., & Spencer-Harper, L. (2017). Experience of PTG in UK veterans with PTSD: A qualitative study. *Royal Army Medical Corps, 163*, 171–176.

Pargament, K. I., & Ano, G. G. (2006). Spiritual resources and struggles in coping with medical illness. *Southern Medical Journal, 99*(10), 1161–1162. https://doi.org/10.1097/01.smj.0000242847.40214.b6

Park, C. L. (2010). Making sense of the meaning literature: An integrative review of 36 studies. *Psychol Bulletin, 136*(2): 61–79.

Park, C. L., Cohen, L. H., & Murch, R. (1996). Assessment and prediction of stress-related growth. *Journal of Personality, 64*, 71–105.

Roberts, C., & Hyatt, L. (2019). *The dissertation journey.* Sage.

Sawyer, A., Ayer, S., Young, D., Bradley, R., & Smith, H. (2012). Posttraumatic growth after childbirth. *Psychology & Health, 27*(3), 362–377.

Shuwiekh, H., Kira, I. A., & Ashby, J. S. (2018). What are the personality and trauma dynamics that contribute to posttraumatic growth? *International Journal of Stress Management, 25*(2), 181–194.

Soo, H., & Sherwin, K. A. (2015). Rumination, psychological distress, and post-traumatic growth in women diagnosed with breast cancer. *Psychooncology, 24*(1), 70–79. https://doi.org/10.1002/pon.3596

Tedeschi, R., & Calhoun, L. (1995). *Trauma and transformation: Growth in the aftermath of suffering.* Sage.

Tedeschi, R., & Calhoun, L. (1996). The posttraumatic growth inventory: Measuring the positive legacy of trauma. *Journal of Traumatic Stress, 9*(3), 455–472.

Tedeschi, R., & Calhoun, L. (2004). Posttraumatic growth: Conceptual foundations and empirical evidence. *Psychological Inquiry, 15*(1), 1–18.

Tennen, H., & Afleck, G. (2009). Assessing positive life change: In search of meticulous methods. In C. L. Park, S. C. Lechner, M. H. Antoni, & A. L. Stanton (Eds.), *Medical illness and positive life change: Can crisis lead to personal transformation?* (pp. 31–49). American Psychological Association.

Tsai, J., Sippel, L., Mota, N., Southwick, S., & Pietrak, R. (2016). Longitudinal cause of posttraumatic growth among U.S. military veterans: Results from the national health and resilience in veterans study. *Depression and Anxiety, 33*(3), 9–18.

# 3

# POSTTRAUMATIC GROWTH AND THE LOSS OF A HUSBAND OR LONGTIME PARTNER

The death of a spouse or longtime partner can be one of the most stressful of all life events. In 2018, there were 11.4 million women widowed as compared to 3.47 million men widowed in the United States (Roberts & Adams, 2018). Widowhood is more common in older adults. In the United States, 14.7% of men and 42.9% of women aged 75 and older are widowed (King et al., 2019). Becoming a widow at an earlier age forces a woman to go through changes that she has not expected to make for many years. These deaths usually commence a dramatic and significant change in one's life compared to before the loss. Some deaths occur suddenly without warning, whereas others follow a gradual decline due to a chronic or terminal illness. Unanticipated widowhood can be the result of accidents, sudden cardiopulmonary or neurological events, and acts of violence.

To be able to function after a spouse's death, one needs to adapt to this change. Bereavement is the process of experiencing and assimilating the loss, whereas grief is the emotional response to the loss, and mourning signifies the actions and manner of expressing one's grief (Stroebe et al., 2007). Grief is an intensely personal response to the loss of a loved one. People respond to the loss of a spouse or longtime partner in their unique way and experience the process of grieving, mourning, and coping with the loss on their personal and unique timetable and trajectory (Kenen, 2021). Grief is primarily shaped by culture, social context, and the nature of the relationship between the grieving individual and the deceased. Mourning practices usually reflect the cultural and religious norms of the bereaved person. Bereavement, grieving, and mourning are complex and multifaceted areas of human experience (Stroebe et al., 2007).

**What Does the Research Tell Us?**

Most research about widowhood has focused on widows who are 60 years of age or older. Very little has been written about midlife widows between 35 and 60 years of age. Even less has been studied or written about widows under 35 years of age. However, with the long duration of US involvement in the wars in Iraq and Afghanistan, there is most likely a sizable cadre of young widows. Most literature about widowhood has centered

DOI: 10.4324/9781003456650-3

on physical and mental health, financial security, bereavement issues, and social support. Research suggests that all of these aforementioned factors are important variables in life and adjustment to widowhood (Ramadas & Kuttichira, 2013). Which of these variables will play a more prominent role for a widow depends on her unique situation, marital history, and life history (Kenen, 2021).

### Research on Health Risks for Widows

The death of a husband or longtime partner has been associated with a greater risk of developing physical and mental health issues, especially during the first year after the death (Ramadas & Kuttichira, 2013). Bereavement of widowhood has been linked to impaired immune function, neuroendocrine changes, and sleep disorders, as well as increased alcohol, prescription drug or illegal drug use, unintentional weight loss, malnutrition, and an increase in hospitalization (DiGiacomo, Davidson, et al., 2013; Mostofsky et al., 2012). The research literature describes various aspects of psychological functioning after the death of a husband or longtime partner (Kristiansen, Kjær, et al., 2019a, 2019b). Death has been found to increase the surviving woman's vulnerability to depression regardless of the mode of death. Widows who seemed most vulnerable to depression were those who lacked social support and who experienced a substantial loss of income related to the death (Kenen, 2021; Scannell-Desch, 2005a, 2005b). Psychological symptoms such as depression, anxiety, and guilt may result from losing a person in a close relationship (Hansford & Jobson, 2021). In addition, emotional and environmental stressors may cause the body to become more susceptible to physical illness (Das, 2013). Thus, the loss of a spouse or partner affects almost every domain of life and has a significant impact on well-being—psychological, physical, social, spiritual, and economic (Bennett et al., 2010; Bennett & Soulsby, 2012). These changes can result in serious illness and even death (Moon et al., 2011).

Some researchers found that women whose husbands suffered from a serious chronic or terminal illness and were forewarned of their impending loss suffered pre-loss depression that did not significantly increase after the death (Guldin et al., 2013). This suggests that anticipatory grieving may play a role in mediating depression following spousal death. Other research suggests that the role of religion, spirituality, and improved end-of-life care can mediate the severity of depressive symptoms (Asai et al., 2013).

### Research on the Financial Impact of Loss

The financial aspects of the loss of a spouse or longtime partner have not received much attention in the research literature. Lancaster and Johnson (2020) reported that research studies found a 33% decline in household wealth during the two years following a husband's death. DiGiacomo et al. (2015) reported a similar decline in household income. DiGiacomo et al. (2013a) reported that widows had lower net worth, fewer financial assets, and a larger percentage of assets invested in housing than similar-aged widowers and married women. DiGiacomo et al. (2015) found that widows had significantly lower wealth holdings than their married or divorced counterparts. Widowhood is much more likely to cause financial stress and hardships for women than for men owing to continued gender disparities in salaries, work histories, and pensions or retirement plans. Some widows postponed entering the workforce to raise children or left the workforce early to care for children or aging parents.

DiGiacomo et al. (2015) longitudinally studied the widowhood experiences of 21 community-dwelling widows over the age of 65. This study aimed to describe women's experiences in the period soon after their husband's death, including their financial issues and concerns, and how these experiences impacted the transition to widowhood late in life. These widows reported over and over again their unmet needs for assistance with administrative, financial, and legal issues immediately following their husbands' death and potentially for years afterward. The widow's lack of familiarity with financial instruments, and the absence of knowledgeable support with financial and legal issues added significant stress for these women during the grieving period. Complex administrative processes with banks, insurance companies, stock and bond companies, and pension administrators, as well as at times insensitive interactions with "gatekeepers" at these institutions contributed to widows' distress, anxiety, and demoralization. Several widows reported that the assumption of household financial management was the most difficult part of coping with their husband's death (DiGiacomo et al., 2015; DiGiacomo, Lewis, et al., 2013b).

## Research on Social Support for Widows

Social support from others is a positive, protective factor for people who have experienced trauma (Hansford & Jobson, 2021). Perceived social support was the most consistent predictor of psychological adjustment to widowhood articulated in the research literature. Some studies found widows' families to be the most important source of support following spousal death. Other studies emphasized that families may not be emotionally available to provide empathetic support for the widow and that other venues of social support may need to be explored (Doherty & Scannell-Desch, 2021; Mark et al., 2018). Additional sources of support may include widows' support groups sponsored by hospitals and religious institutions, hospice organizations, or the Internet. Eshbaugh (2008) and Kenen (2021) conclude that widows' families may offer initial support after the death, but support from friends and peers may become the primary support over time.

Scannell-Desch (2005a, 2005b) conducted a qualitative study of ten mid-life widows between the ages of 35 and 60 years. The study aimed to ascertain descriptions of supportive and non-supportive experiences following the death of their husbands. Findings indicated that listening was the most supportive behavior of others. These women found that friends who simply listened and did not try to give advice or control the conversation were most helpful and supportive. These widows also found that those who offered practical support, such as picking the children up at school, mowing the lawn, fixing the dishwasher, and doing grocery shopping offered hands-on support that was most appreciated. Nonsupportive behaviors included people who tried to give unsolicited advice, practiced avoidance and distancing, and made irritating remarks, such as "You are young, you'll find love again" or "You are lucky you don't have children."

## Our Study Themes

As researchers and authors, we conducted a study in 2020 to assess posttraumatic growth in 14 widows. We want to share several themes that emerged from our data analysis. We believe this will help to frame the widows' stories and shed additional light on the meaning of their experiences and possible journeys to posttraumatic growth. The themes are (1) anticipated loss, (2) unanticipated loss, (3) a new depth of compassion and empathy, (4) my strength grew over time, and (5) my view of myself changed.

## Our Study Methods

Our methods for recruiting widows for our study included the use of purposive and snowball sampling. Purposive sampling means that the researcher deliberately chooses a sample to study that most likely will provide information that will answer the research questions. Snowball sampling is a recruitment technique where existing study subjects recruit future subjects from among people they are acquainted with. Thus, the sample group is said to grow like a rolling snowball. As the sample grows in the number of people, enough data are gathered to be useful for the research study. Study participants were recruited through the investigators' nursing network, which comprised faculty and clinical colleagues at affiliated hospitals. Institutional Review Board approval was granted by the university where the first author was employed. Inclusion criteria were women who identified themselves as a widow for at least five years; the ability to read, write, and speak English; the ability to recall the experience of a spouse's or partner's death; and willingness to discuss the experience. We decided that a five-year period of time between the death and the research interview was a reasonable interval to allow for adjustment. Potential participants who met inclusion criteria were mailed a letter explaining the study and the concept of PTG. A consent form and return mailing envelope were included for those interested in participating in the study. Fourteen consent forms and demographic information sheets were completed and returned. After written consent was obtained, an email was sent to schedule an interview at the participant's convenience. Data were collected from Fall 2020 through Fall 2021. A mental health nurse practitioner was available for debriefing if any participant became upset or felt uncomfortable during or after the interview. None of the participants needed debriefing or counseling.

## Theme: Anticipated Loss

### Lucinda and Terrence

"My husband died at age 41 after a long battle with alcoholism. I think his problem with alcohol began in his late twenties and continued until his death. It ended up being a peaceful death in the hospital, and it was a relief from his suffering. It was a relief for me, too, because the problem had continued for at least 10–12 years, and it got worse with every passing year. It was a long and difficult illness that affected me and our three children as well. Terrence deteriorated in every possible way: mentally, physically, spiritually, and character-wise. It was very hard to watch over time. It not only affected his life but also my life and the lives of our three children. He was not there to offer parental support. I had to do an awful lot of things by myself and for my children."

**Lucinda** continued, "Over the years, Terrence kept getting worse. He must have been in and out of at least ten treatment programs paid for by his employer. He had a good executive position and traveled quite a bit. But the traveling covered up the extent of the problem because he drank on airplanes and in hotel rooms away from his family. Even in his office, he kept a bottle in the bottom drawer of his desk, and his secretary either covered up for him or ignored the problem. I'm sure co-workers did, too. He worked for a very large company with offices throughout the US and the world."

**Lucinda** recalled, "I was with Terrence when he died. He would usually call about once a week to check in with me and the kids. Many times, he didn't make a lot of sense on the phone; he often talked gibberish. Even when the kids went years without seeing him, he did call. Then, one weekend there was no phone call, and I became worried and called his parents in New England. They had not heard from him. Later, I got a call from his aunt, and she said he was in this hospital nearby where we lived in the Midwest. I went there early on Sunday morning with a friend of mine and we found him. He was dying. Over the years, he had endured a lot of falls and had brain damage. When I saw him, he was attached to a lot of machines. I stayed with him, and I think he knew I was there. It was a very peaceful death. I remember asking the nursing staff to have a Catholic priest come and give him the Last Rites because he was a Catholic throughout his life. It took a while for them to get a priest, but in the meantime, I think five or six ministers came by to bless him. I think we hit all the Protestant denominations. Finally, the priest arrived, and he was wonderful. After Terrence passed away, the priest told me to go and get some peace in my life."

### Cora and Brad

"I always knew Brad would pass away because of his health problems, but we didn't know that it would be so soon. He had a cardiac arrest while on the list for a heart transplant. He knew that he had heart problems for a very long time. They thought he had a hole in his heart as a child. Later they said he had cardiomyopathy. The disease was called ISH or something like that. They explained it to me, but I don't remember the details because I don't have a medical background. When Brad was younger, he lived the way he wanted to and drank and smoked cigarettes. He ate whatever food he wanted to eat. I guess what I'm trying to say is that he didn't follow the doctor's advice. His death was hard on the family because we had four sons ranging in age from 11 to 19."

### Lydia and Mike

"In 2007 my husband, Mike, wasn't feeling well. He was having a loss of appetite, indigestion, and mid-back pain, and had lost about 15 pounds. He was diagnosed with pancreatic cancer, and three weeks later he was gone. It was a total shock. I was like a zombie. I went through my life like a robot doing everything I did, but not feeling anything. Two months after he passed away, my mother passed away. So, I was in double zombie land. I kept on working and having a life, but not paying attention to it, just going through the motions. A year later in 2008, I was diagnosed with breast cancer. I had bilateral mastectomies and implants. I went through chemo. Two months later my daughter was diagnosed with breast cancer. She had a double mastectomy and chemo, but her chemo was worse than mine. She now has metastatic breast cancer. My life has been on automatic pilot since 2007."

### Marilyn and Dave

**Marilyn** recalled, "I was in my thirties. I think I was 34, and Dave was three years older than me, so he was 37, and we lived in Italy at the time because Dave was in the US Air Force. We were assigned over there, and Dave came in from jogging one day. He went out for a jog and came back and said that he had fallen. He was not sure what happened. So, we patched him up, and he said that he didn't feel right, so we went to the on-base clinic that morning. We had Kenny, and he was probably two years old. I was out of the Air Force but had just taken a job as a civilian RN at the base clinic. I was approved to start in a few weeks. I had hired an Italian nanny, and I was excited about that, thinking that I'd have this bi-lingual child."

"We ended up getting an appointment at the Naples clinic, which was maybe an hour-and-a-half to two-hour drive. It was a Navy clinic in Naples. We had a morning appointment, and we had a camper at the time, and we took that thing all over the place. We had a dog, too, so I had to put the dog in, and then Kenny and off we went to Naples. They did an MRI and said, "We think Dave may have had a minor stroke, so we want to keep him overnight." So, I stayed in the camper with Kenny and the dog. Then, they determined that they needed to fly Dave up to Landstuhl Army Hospital in Germany. They med-evac-ed him up there. They sent a C-9 aircraft, and he was the only patient on it. I appreciated that. It must have been considered urgent because it was the middle of the morning when they picked him up. I had to drive the camper back from Naples. I never liked that drive anyway, especially when everyone had mini-cars and I had this big old camper."

"I got back to San Vito where we lived, and I'm a nervous wreck. As a nurse, I am asking all the right questions, and they couldn't come up with anything because they are a small clinic. They got me a flight up to Landstuhl, and they told me to pack for 30 days. So, I packed for 30 days for me and Kenny and some of Dave's stuff. When I got there, they had already done a bunch of tests and determined that it was a brain tumor. So, they were going to send us back stateside and they asked us where we wanted to go."

"We had been stationed in San Antonio, Texas, earlier in our careers but picked the east coast because we had family there, so it was Walter Reed Army Medical Center. They med-evac-ed us up there. I remember that we flew in on Halloween. We all flew together, sitting in regular seats on a C-141 Starlifter. Poor little Kenny had earplugs and headphones on. It was a long flight for him."

"Dave's parents met us at the USO Greeting Center at Andrews Air Force Base, and we ended up going over to Walter Reed Army Medical Center together. They did more testing and a biopsy. They send everything to the Armed Forces Institute of Pathology. We eventually ended up in Alabama, where we had been before being reassigned to Italy. They sent the pathology report to the University of Alabama Medical Center in Birmingham. They said it was an oligodendroglioma, which was a better prognosis than what they had originally said at Walter Reed. The doctors at Walter Reed said, "Go do what you want, basically you don't have a lot of time.""

"So, I'm dealing with his parents that are not accepting this very well and me with my medical knowledge having worked on a neuro floor in my career knowing that this all was not very good. Dave ended up being medically discharged, which happened while we were still in Germany just because it was a better outcome financially and medically for the family. It was better to medically retire someone than to leave them on active duty. Dave pinned on his Major rank in the hospital, and we ended up back stateside in Alabama eventually."

"He got all of his treatment at Walter Reed Medical Center in Washington, DC. We spent a lot of time driving back and forth from Alabama. He had radiation for six or eight weeks. We'd come up to New Jersey and visit with my family on weekends and then go back. We stayed in base housing when he was getting his treatment, and then we went back to Alabama to be closer to his parents. He was an Alabama resident, and overall that ended up being a good thing because both of my kids were eligible for a free college education later. We also used the VA up in Birmingham for some treatments."

"I had a surprise pregnancy with Bobby. I was not expecting that and delivered in Montgomery so Bobby is an Alabama baby. I stayed there until Dave passed away and then came up to New Jersey. We stayed with my Dad because my Mom ended up passing away six months before my husband did. It was three years from diagnosis till when Dave died. He passed away at 41 years of age. So, we ended up in New Jersey, and I've spent the last 25 years there."

### Christy and Marty

**Christy** reported, "My husband died of cancer nine years ago. Marty was my best friend, my soulmate, my confidant, and a wonderful husband and father. It was a second marriage for both of us. We both had adult children from our first marriages. We met many years ago in the Army Reserve. He was a laboratory technician who went back to college to become a registered nurse. I was a registered nurse. We had so much in common, and our personalities gravitated toward each other. We both had first marriages long behind us."

"He had head and neck cancer diagnosed and treated with surgery and radiation, but it recurred several years later and became metastatic. The Army let him stay on with a profile for US deployments only, whereas I was worldwide deployable. Shortly after he died, his youngest son got into some trouble and committed suicide. So, I had to deal with my husband's death and the death of his son, whom we were very close to. These were mind-numbing experiences. I just had to put 'one foot in front of the other' day after day to keep from drowning. It was like being in a hurricane or tornado and struggling to find shelter or a safe place. I had one close girlfriend who helped and became my sounding board to keep me from going crazy. When I called, she always came to the house."

"During our marriage, I was deployed to Germany for six months and later to Iraq for six months. I enjoyed both of my deployments, but I worried about his health while I was gone. Looking back, his health was very stable during both of my deployments. I knew he worried about my safety while I was in Iraq. I was afraid it would take a toll on him and his health, however, he did fine while I was gone. He was deployed to Florida and Alabama while I was deployed in Iraq. We both had busy and productive jobs while on active duty. He liked what he was doing and I liked what I was doing. We were an adventurous couple, who liked to work hard for causes we believed in. We were both very patriotic and believed in the ideals of our country and the US Army."

### Paige and Ben

"My husband called me at work. He said that he wasn't feeling well. He had pain in his left side. I told him to call 911, which he did because there were no neighbors around. They admitted him to the hospital because they wanted to do a bunch of tests. They concluded that his adrenal gland had burst. He was discharged from the hospital on Sunday night and was referred to a specialist. I think it was an endocrinologist. While at the hospital, they asked a lot of questions about a melanoma he had removed in the past. It was a few years ago. Finally, the endocrine doctor showed up at 7:00 PM. He had Ben walk across the floor and watched him. Then we were sent home with plans to see a cancer specialist for more tests. So, on Tuesday, we had an appointment with an oncologist. On July 1, the test results showed cancer. It was mentioned a few times that they did not know why the adrenal gland burst. Ben passed away on August 5. It was unexpected, and it hit me like a ton of bricks. The original thought was that this cancer was related to melanoma and that it spread over time. They first said that the median survival rate was 18 months. They mentioned that the preliminary research at Yale was promising. Ben had a PET scan and an appointment at Yale was scheduled."

**Paige** recalled, "In mid-July, the oncologist told us that Ben had metastasis to the brain. We suspected that this was not good and that is when our son Jim came from Australia. We were hoping that Ben had 18 months. He was so brave, too. The oncologist noticed that Ben had a shuffling gait, but neither of us was sure how long he had it. Every day there was something new. I finally asked in frustration, 'How long are we talking about?' Now, the oncologist said about 10 months rather than 18 months. I was working full-time in New York City with a long commute each way from Connecticut. Sometimes I was able to work from home one day a week. It was very stressful with my work situation and the long commute. Our son, Jim, stayed at home with Ben while I worked. I asked my boss about more opportunities to work from home. My immediate manager had less management experience and did not say, 'Take whatever time that you need,' which made my situation extremely stressful. There was so much uncertainty. I stayed home with Ben until Jim arrived from Australia. I found out that family medical leave can be taken in increments. Initially, I thought it was 60 or 90 days of unpaid leave, but I learned that the law allows you to take time off in increments as needed. In all of this, hope is so important. You can't give up. Different therapies were recommended such as a few different kinds of radiation. A specialist at another hospital was recommended for a specific type of radiation, but I can't remember exactly."

"Ben was a brilliant man! He loved to read and was very intellectual. He ended up having radiation at the first hospital. It was tough. Our son Jim took him while I was at work. Ben became a different person. He would go outside to have a cigarette and become confused as he came back into the house. Sometimes he seemed angry and agitated and his personality changed. It was very stressful because there was so much uncertainty, and you know you are going to lose someone you love shortly. Then, there are obligations at work. I felt pulled in so many different directions. I looked to the doctor for advice about Ben's behavior at home, which became questionable. I remember one horrible night at home. He was agitated, angry, and confused. I knew I needed to take off from work. It was looking bad and becoming more difficult. Everything happened so fast. I remember talking to a male RN from the VNA. When he was leaving the house, he said that sometimes the patient may not want to remain home. He used the word 'hospice.' Ben agreed. In private, the nurse told me, 'This could happen sooner than you think.' He said to contact hospice ASAP. Everything became a blur to me; then he went into hospice care at a nearby long-term care facility. It was very close to where we lived. I met with my boss and said I need to leave. I took two weeks' vacation starting on Friday, July 25. I met with hospice, and the palliative care team, and visited Ben every day. I could see that he was getting weaker and losing his hair. I brought our dog Pepper to visit him. Pepper was Ben's dog, and we had a wonderful visit that Monday night. Ben seemed worried, and I asked him 'What are you worried about?' He replied, 'Missing you.' The next day, our son Jim insisted that I get a new car. He was concerned because my car was getting old. While at the car dealer, I got a call that Ben had passed away. It was all so fast!"

### Barbara and Jack

"My husband died at the age of 57 when he had his third heart attack. I was in my late forties, but I was prepared in a way because his second heart attack was a very bad one. After his second heart attack, Jack was in the ICU for more than a month. He was on a ventilator and was in a coma. I knew from the doctors that if he had another one, it would probably kill him. I never thought he would go home again, but he lived for about five months in a rehabilitation facility. Unfortunately, our health insurance only paid for the first month because he was brain-damaged and not considered a viable rehabilitation candidate. Our insurance did not pay for the custodial care provided after the first month. Those months were agony for me. I was so stressed emotionally and financially. My brothers and sisters lived over 500 miles from us, and they could not help in a practical sense but called frequently to get an update on Jack. Not only was I preparing for my husband to die, but I was facing thousands of dollars in medical bills. When he finally passed away, it was kind of a relief to me because he was no longer suffering and I was not incurring more debt from a futile situation. His death was peaceful in that he just went to sleep and stopped breathing."

### Louise and Don

"My husband died from pancreatic cancer. He had surgery twice. It took eight hours of surgery the second time because my husband was a big man and they had a lot of scar tissue to cut through from the first surgery. I'd take him for chemo after the two surgeries. Sometimes I'd just take him in for an IV to get hydrated. One day I noticed he had little blisters all over his body. The doctor said all of his systems were shutting down."

"One day he was doing very badly. So, the doctor said I could bring him to his office and he'd call an ambulance to take him to the hospital. He said that if I drove him to the hospital, he'd be stuck in the ER for a long time. The doctor said if we came to his office, he could do a direct admission, which would bypass the ER. So, I got him in the car and drove him to the doctor's office and then he was admitted directly to the hospital."

"In the weeks before he died, I'd take him to Great Kills on Staten Island to see the boats because he loved boats and the water. It was so hard to get him down the stairs. He was a big man and 6 foot 2 inches. We'd watch the boats for 15 minutes, and then he'd ask if we could go home because he was so tired. I'd do anything he wanted to do. I never let him see me cry, but I cried a lot in another room when he was sleeping. I could not let him see that this was killing me. I had to be strong. When one of his friends would come by, he'd relieve me for 40 minutes so I could go to the grocery store. Then I come home and sit in the driveway outside the house and cry."

"The last time he came home from the hospital, he said, 'No more chemo.' He lasted about two weeks. Hospice came, but they couldn't do much for him in the end because he was so weak. We talked a lot during those two weeks. He told me to go on with my life and not accept an insurance check. He told me his last wishes were for immediate cremation. He didn't want a viewing or anything like that. He was just the best, the most wonderful person. He smiled a lot and had kind words for everyone. He'd make people laugh. He made people around him feel good. He was 61 when he died."

### Patty and Drew

**Patty** recalled, "We had a magical life together; in that, we both needed each other. I was a stepchild and came second to everybody. He was the first son in a long line of sons, and he was not appreciated either by his family. Neither of us was educated, but we helped each other grow. Later, we both got formal education. My husband went to college as a young adult and got his engineering degree. After he got his education and the children were in school, I went to college to get my degree. We had 68 very fulfilling years together. We moved to New Jersey to be closer to our children after he had several mini-strokes. He lived a long, happy, and productive life. Drew passed away six years ago from a final stroke after 68 years of marriage. I am 94 now."

## Theme: Unanticipated loss

### Clarice and Dan

"On Nov 12, 2005, we were cleaning up the yard. Dan said, 'I'm not even going to clean up the whole yard today because I'm a little tired.' But then he got going and said to himself, 'I'm just going to finish this.' I said, "Okay, whatever you want to do." I didn't think too much about it. So, I'm inside working on a community history project, and I'm standing in the kitchen and I can't see where Dan was working because Mitch had parked his friend's big truck outside blocking my view earlier in the day. So, all of a sudden, this woman came banging on the door. She said, 'Quick, quick, call 911—there is a man on the ground in front of your house.' So, I thought it was a man going on a walk by my house. She said, 'You've got to come outside with your phone right away.' So, I had the portable phone in my hand, and I went outside. And, oh my God, Dan was on the ground near the lawnmower. It still wasn't registering. I called 911 and gave them the information. And then just like everything went into slow motion. I can remember everything vividly, but it seemed like it took forever for the ambulance to get there. I remember the fire engine came down the road like it was going five miles an hour. I got down and was going to start CPR, but one of my neighbors came over and got down and started CPR. In my mind, it was like, 'What is happening?' I got down on my knees and put my hands on him and prayed, really prayed. And God said to me, 'No, it's his time.' I get chills thinking about it, but it was so clear. So, I stood there and I thought, 'Whoa.' I called a close friend of ours; he is a physician's assistant in Boston. He came over right away so he could help the fireman. I called my children just to tell them what was up. Two were on their way home and got there when the ambulance was still there. Our son, Mitch, said to him, 'How does it look?' and he said, 'It doesn't look good.' He had already died. I had a little bit of hope, I heard some noise and thought he was trying to breathe. But it was what you call the 'death rattle.' I knew he was gone because of my experience of praying and the answer I got. We had friends that took us to the hospital. People from our church called other people from our church. I think the whole church showed up at the ER, and the staff let them all in. It was just incredible. Everyone was just hysterical because Dan was an elder at the church. They always called him the 'approachable elder.' He loved everyone and was so good with the kids. Everyone was just devastated. Everyone was all over the halls and waiting area. Then the doctor asked me and Mitch and Ellen to come into the room where Dan was. They were still working on him, but I knew he was gone. I knew that at the house. But they have to do this. They tried and they tried in the ambulance and up to the hospital, and I am grateful for this. Then he said to his staff, can anyone think of anything else we can do? Everyone said 'No.' He looked at me and said, 'Then it is time for us to call it.' And I said 'Okay.' He had that tube sticking out of his throat. I hate those tubes. I said please get that thing out of there, and he removed it. He then asked if I wanted an autopsy. And this is something I regret. I said 'No.' But now with what has happened to his two brothers, I wish I had an autopsy so the family could know more. The doctor told me Dan had a massive heart attack and that is why he went so quickly. I remember all these people came in, and I thought, 'I don't know what to do.' I said, 'Will someone please tell me what to do?'"

"It is expected and it is unexpected. This was so unexpected. I think I was in shock. I have to say I felt like there was a protective bubble around me. I think God gives us a protective bubble around us so we can handle certain things. The bubble helps you deal with things later. It was crazy. A friend of mine went and got my parents. My father is looking at me like, 'Why aren't you crying.' And I'm not a crier. Tears didn't come. I was broken inside but tears didn't come. I've always been that way and I don't know why. It was awful. But I have such a strong faith. I know that God is sovereign, and I know that this was part of his plan. God knew this the day Dan was born. This was his time. Mitch said the same thing to me. This was Dad's time. That gave me such peace when Mitch said that. Later, I called up neighbors and said, 'Come over, I want to share good memories of Dan.' And they came over, and we all talked. People from the church and the neighborhood came over and shared memories and stories of Dan, and that was so soothing for me. He was loved. I don't know why I did that; that was the evening that he died. It was as soon as I got home from the hospital. I wanted to talk about Dan. Right before that, he was so worried about me. I was getting diverticulitis all the time and was in and out of the hospital. He said that morning, 'It is chilly and I want you to stay in the house. I don't want you to get sick.' We didn't know his heart was having trouble. He had been complaining the last couple of months of being tired and getting leg cramps. He also had some shortness of breath. I had told him to make the first appointment he could in primary care because the doctor he saw was a cardiologist. He died on Nov 12, and the first appointment he could get was the first week of December. However, I don't beat myself up or go there. It was his time, and this was part of God's plan. If one of his brothers had a heart problem first, we would have been alerted more and pushed for an earlier appointment or gone to the ER."

The next day: "My father-in-law was living with us. Someone called and said when do you want him out, I said 'today,' I can't deal with this. You need to come and get him today. I was so worried something would happen to him. I tried to keep him from seeing Dan on the ground, I put him in the car and said to stay there. One of the neighbors then took him into the house, stayed with him, and explained to him what happened."

### Jocelyn and Liam

"My husband died in 1988. My kids were four years old and two years old, and they both had birthdays coming up. It was pretty sudden. He died of a heart attack in his sleep. Looking back, it is kind of a blur because, with a two-year-old and a four-year-old, you have to wake up every day and keep doing things. To be honest, I was probably on automatic pilot for a couple of weeks, yet I remember that day because he died at his mother's house. He was taking a nap downstairs. He had brought the two kids over with him, and I was supposed to come over later. His mother said to the kids, 'Let's go wake up your father.' So, it was the two kids trying to wake him up. And when he didn't wake up, my mother-in-law knew something was wrong. I was on the phone with my mother, and the operator broke into the line saying that there was an emergency call for me. It was from my mother-in-law's house, but it was her neighbor on the phone. He's a retired oral surgeon. They had called the ambulance and all that. It took me longer than usual to drive over because there was a lot of road construction. When I got there the ambulance had already left but the police were still there. They didn't take Liam to the hospital because they realized that he had been dead for a while. The call was very scary when the operator broke into the line. Liam didn't have a history of heart problems, but his father died the same way. He had been napping for about 1 1/2 hours but must have died at the beginning of the nap according to the ambulance people who tried to revive him. His body was still there when I arrived because they didn't take him to the hospital and they were waiting for the medical examiner to come to the house. My mother and father came over, too. One neighbor had the kids at her house coloring pictures. They had not realized what had happened because they were so young. When my mother-in-law realized something was wrong with Liam, she screamed, and their neighbor Mike came over immediately, and his wife took the kids back to their house. The police stayed until the medical examiner arrived because they can't leave until the body is taken out of the house."

"I was in a fog and my parents took the kids back to their house. My brothers and sisters were there. My sister, Kayla, and I were the only ones that had kids. I was only 30 years old and Liam was 40 years old, but there were heart problems on his father's side of the family. It was a very traumatic day. It was pretty difficult for me. Then, later I had to tell the kids and they didn't understand."

### Maura and Wesley

"My husband died at 28 years of age in a one-car motor vehicle accident. The state police think he fell asleep at the wheel on a long drive. He was a graduate student driving from San Francisco to Los Angeles by himself. He veered off the road at night, going down an embankment; the car flipped over several times, and he died on impact. At the time, I was on a Caribbean cruise with my older sister. They could not reach me on the ship because this was 1978. So, my mother had to tell me when I arrived home. I was in shock for a long time. My husband had been my college boyfriend. We had been married for five years, and we were hoping to start a family during his second year of graduate school."

### Marissa and Rob

"Rob was my first husband, and he was 27 years old. He was a long-distance runner. He went out with the guys the night before his last race. They were all runners. That morning, we got up and got the two kids dressed and went to the town where the race was scheduled. We then met his friends there. Rob ran during his freshmen year of college and always ran for exercise. He worked for IBM and had his Ph.D. in chemistry. So, we watched the race, and it was a half marathon. After a while, I started to see his IBM friends come across the finish line and no Rob to be seen. I asked some of his friends if they saw him, and at first, they joked around and said, 'Some lady whistled at him and he went into her house.' Then when more time passed and still no Rob, we all started getting concerned. We started asking the race officials, and they said that someone had collapsed on the run and was taken by ambulance to a hospital. When we asked what hospital, they said they didn't know. So, I went to a phone booth and started calling hospitals. They had taken him to a community hospital. When I got there, he was conscious but couldn't make any sense when he tried to talk. It was all garbled sounds. The people in the ER told me they didn't exactly know what was wrong with him. They said it was probably a drug reaction and he had maybe taken LSD. The doctors introduced themselves, 'I am a doctor so and so, and this is a doctor so and so, and we think this is some type of drug reaction.' I and his IBM friends said there is no way Rob took any drugs. They said at IBM we do complete physicals and all sorts of blood tests, and there is no way Rob was on any drugs. I said, 'For God's sake, he was running a race. Druggies are not athletes, they are not long-distance runners, this is crazy.' Then they shot him up with Valium to calm him down. The IBM couple took my children back to their house. So, then I was there by myself. The hospital people started acting erratically. They said I had to have someone come and sit with him because he was so restless and out of it. It was terrible, and they were just horrible. They restrained him, which drove me crazy. They tied him down. So, then they put a catheter in him, and then I noticed blood in his urine. That's essentially what happened, he got DIC (disseminated intravascular coagulopathy). When he was in the ambulance, they iced him, they did everything they were supposed to do to cool him down. He went from heat exhaustion to heatstroke and then eventually went into DIC. Once he got to the hospital, they stopped icing him, and that is when he went from heat exhaustion to heatstroke. They didn't continue icing him in the ER, because they thought he was on drugs. So, all of it was preventable. They shipped him to a medical center by ambulance and put him in intensive care. The doctors there knew what happened when I told them the story. A doctor came in, and I was all by myself, and the doctor asked me if I ever thought about my philosophy of death. I couldn't believe this, I said 'No, I'm only 27 years old.' He said I think you need to think about this because it is very unlikely your husband is going to survive this. Then they called in a surgeon, and the surgeon said he wouldn't touch him with a ten-foot pole. He lasted for three days in their ICU and then he died. They couldn't do anything for him. They said the only reason he lasted three days was that he had a very strong heart. He was all bloated with blood from the DIC. I think it was a real miserable death, but that is what happened."

### Laila and Jim

**Laila** recalled, "I was in a master's program, and I was up late getting some work done. My husband fell asleep on the couch, which was not unusual. When I went to bed around 2:00 AM, he was still there, and I decided to just let him sleep there. I didn't want to awaken him. When I got up the next morning, he was still asleep on the couch but was in an uncomfortable-looking position, so I went over to him. I could not wake him up. He had died. My daughter was home from college, and I yelled upstairs for her. She thought I was just trying to get her up and out of bed, and she started yelling at me. She was very upset when she found out the real reason why I was calling for her. My middle son was in Alaska with the Army. He had just come back from being deployed to Iraq. My older son was working in New York City. So, I had to make those phone calls. It was very difficult, and I was still in shock."

"There was a strong family history of heart problems in my husband's family, but my husband did not have heart problems that we knew about. His father had heart surgery twice. My husband was trying to quit smoking at the time, and he was 58 years old. He was wearing three nicotine patches that I did not know about, but the funeral director told me that. I thought, 'Oh my God he was probably hypotensive because of those patches. You're not supposed to wear more than one at a time. He never told me about that stuff or asked me about it. He just did his own thing. I know that those patches have lots of properties that can cause hypotension. He was trying to quit smoking on his own. He was under a lot of pressure at work in the publishing business, and things were getting more high-tech. There were a lot of changes in the book industry with textbooks and encyclopedias. My husband was also stressed because after his dad died, he took over the family business and lost a court case with a construction company. As a result, his family lost about 200 acres of property. It was a very stressful time for him. It had been a long-drawn-out court battle."

"He died thirteen years ago in March of 2007, which was three months before our 30th anniversary. You know, it is what it is. When he died my kids were grown. My daughter was in college. I had to get my son emergency leave from the Army in Alaska. It was difficult, and I had to contact the American Red Cross and later the police. He was on Army active duty, and they would not fly him home, and the regular airfare was more than $3000. A friend reached out to a legislator to expedite the trip. It's upsetting to talk about this, but I want to tell you the whole story."

### *Joy and Carl*

**Joy** recalled, "I was three months pregnant with my second child. My husband was a chemistry teacher and went to school to set up the lab for his students. He was passionate about teaching and liked to be organized for both class and lab. When he didn't return home by dinner, I called his office at the school, but there was no answer. This was before I had a cell phone. It was 1992. My oldest child was one and a half years old." Joy continued, "I started to get worried when Carl didn't come home. I felt a little angry when he missed dinner. I wondered if he ran into another teacher and maybe they went out for a drink or something. At 10 PM, I called my parents and told them that I was worried. I tried to go to sleep but couldn't fall asleep. Finally, at one in the morning, I called the local police to report that Carl was missing. The police officer who answered the phone told me that you can't file a missing person report until the person has been missing for 24 hours. So, I figured I would do that in the morning if he was still not home. In the morning, I called Carl's best friend and told him what was going on. He said that something must be wrong because Carl wouldn't just not come home. He said that he had not seen or heard from Carl either and that this was very strange. He told me that he would check into it and call me back. About 30 minutes later I got a call from Carl's best friend telling me that I had to come to the school immediately, that Carl had fallen. He said, 'You have to come right now.' So, I went. When I arrived, the EMS was there. Carl had fallen as a result of a massive heart attack. They told me that he died right away and did not suffer. They didn't want me to see him, but I insisted. I was in such shock. I was in a fog for a long time. The only thing that kept me going was my one-and-a-half-year-old daughter and the baby that I was three months pregnant with. I had nine months of nausea and vomiting during this pregnancy. It was probably hyperemesis gravidarum. I had nausea and vomiting also at the beginning of my first pregnancy, but it went away after a few months. During this pregnancy, I had it the whole time. I was so sick and only gained 22 pounds in total. I'm sure it had to do with the sudden loss of my husband. He was only 38 years old, and I was 24 years old. The autopsy said that it was a massive MI (myocardial infarction). They said he died immediately. What got me through the remainder of the pregnancy was a concern for the baby and my other daughter. They kept me going."

## Theme: A New Depth of Compassion and Empathy

**Lucinda** shared, "I have great compassion and empathy for others. I feel that I am encouraging others because I have been through a very difficult experience. There is a way out. You can't let the ETOH abuse take over your life as it has done with your husband. I remember helping a friend who had a daughter that was married to a drug addict. I gave her advice based on my experience. She thanked me and found my words helpful."

**Jocelyn** recalled, "Yes, I have a greater sense of empathy and compassion for people suffering a loss after I experienced my husband's death. It made me understand things much more acutely. As an ICU nurse, I remember a code (cardiac arrest) and a woman crying in the hallway. I remember going up to her and asking her if I could do something for her. Her husband was not old, and she was worried about her children. She did not know my circumstances, but she asked me, 'What should I tell my children?' I said to her, 'Tell them that you love them.' Her situation brought me back to what I had experienced. I wanted to give a simple and heartfelt response. I was not prepared for this situation, and I did not tell her about my loss or my children. Maybe if I had been a widow longer, I would have shared my experience with her. Plus, I didn't know her, but I feel that I answered her question and showed caring and compassion. As a result of my loss and the stress of bringing up children on my own, I feel that I understand more of what people are going through."

**Cora**, whose husband died from heart failure, stated, "I have compassion for people, but I can't say that it increased after my husband's death. With four kids to take care of, I just tried to get through each day. I didn't have any energy left over at the end of the day. I had to focus on what I needed to do to get by."

**Maura** became a widow when her young husband was killed in a car accident. Maura remarked, "I've always been a very empathetic and compassionate person. However, my level of empathy and compassion for others became deeper after Wesley was killed. I felt my sorrow so profoundly. Being a nurse, I now have 'walked in the shoes' of many patients' families, so I can more acutely feel their pain."

**Paige** related, "It's hard not to be more compassionate and altruistic after going through an experience as I did with Ben dying so quickly from cancer. Everything happened so fast. I'm a practical, no-nonsense person. I felt different doing normal things. This is because I lost a part of myself. I had the rug pulled out from under me. I felt things differently. I can understand the experience better after having lived through it."

**Lydia** reported, "My compassion for people increased after I lost my husband. I now do volunteer work at the Society of St. Vincent de Paul to help the poor. I do home visits, and I can tell you these people have so much faith. They may be poor, but they are not at all angry with God for what they don't have. I try my hardest to not be judgmental."

**Marissa**, whose husband died from heat stroke, recalled, "I had enough love and care to give to my family and my kids, but I didn't have any extra to give to anybody else. I knew it, and I knew my limitations."

**Christy**, whose husband died of cancer, remarked, "I have always been a very compassionate person. One of my dreams and plans which I'm currently working on is to establish a home for homeless women veterans. I had talked with my husband about this idea before he died. We see so many homeless veterans living on the streets, being involved in alcohol and drug abuse, being down on their luck, and some are abandoned by their families or don't have families for support and encouragement. The American public thinks of these veterans as men, but there are women veterans in this predicament, too. But we don't hear about them. Some of the women are alone, but others have small children. Many go from temporary shelter to temporary shelter. I want to give them a home for a month, several months, or even a year where they can get the resources and help they need to find a better and more stable life."

**Marilyn**, whose husband died of a brain tumor at 41, stated, "Yes, of course, I'm compassionate and even more so since Dave's passing. I'm a nurse, and compassion is in our nature as nurses. We want to make people better and help those in need. It's the way we are created. It's in our DNA, you either 'got it or you don't.' As nurses, we've all got it and that's why we go into the nursing profession." Marilyn continued, "Once my kids were in school, I got involved more with my church and its efforts to help people in need. As a school nurse, I always looked out for kids that were struggling, whether it be from poverty, neglect, broken homes, or whatever."

**Barbara's** husband died from his third heart attack at 57 years of age. Barbara related, "I've always had empathy for people and their stressful situations. I have always done some volunteer work in a local soup kitchen and supported various church and local outreach activities. Since Jack's death, I believe my depth of compassion for people in need has increased. I joined a widow's support group at a local church after Jack's death. I soon realized many widows had a much more stressful bereavement experience than I had. My heart goes out to these families with young children having to grow up without their Dad and a stay-at-home Mom who now has to find a job."

**Louise**, whose husband died from pancreatic cancer, related, "Yes, I believe I'm much more understanding and compassionate now. People don't know what is in store for them going through the loss of a husband, or a soulmate. I miss him terribly, but I say to myself, 'No one had what we had.' We had such a wonderful life together. Our marriage and relationship were so good and so close."

**Louise** continued, "I live in a 55+ community, so someone is always dying. I try to be there for people alone and people in need. I don't have any regrets; we had a wonderful life but I just wish it was longer. How I was able to move forward was to think about all that was good. I find good memories keep me in a positive frame of mind. I know my husband would be happy that I bought a house and a car all by myself. He'd be proud that I learned how to do these things from him. I learned a lot about financial matters from him. He always knew I was listening to him, but now I've demonstrated that I could put all I learned from him into practice."

**Patty**, who lost her husband to a stroke after 68 years of marriage, related, "I have had a tremendous sense of humility and gratefulness toward my neighbors and friends since Drew's passing. I feel I've grown through my experience of loss, and I try to be worthy of the friends and neighbors who have helped me, and I am grateful. My mission is to give back to people and to help as many people as I can. I try to reach out to people who need help, or are lonely and need company. God has given me so much over the years, and I see myself as someone who wants to and is willing to serve to help others who are having a rough time. My life has been far more perfect than I could ever dream."

**Laila**, whose husband died from a cardiac arrhythmia while taking a nap, recounted, "I have always had empathy for people in the throes of poverty, disenfranchisement, addiction, mental challenges, and single parenthood. Even though I lost my husband at a very early age, I still understand that my lot in life is better than many people."

**Joy** lost her husband to a massive heart attack at the age of 38. Joy recalled, "Yes, I've always considered myself a compassionate person. I have always helped out in my community and through my church. I am Catholic, and we always donated to Catholic Charities. We also donated clothing to Goodwill. My husband was a volunteer fireman within our community. We lived our faith and gave to others less fortunate."

## Theme: My Strength Grew over Time

**Lucinda** lost her 41-year-old husband to complications from alcoholism. Lucinda stated, "I see my life as a 'triumph.' It was like our priest said, 'Go and find peace,' and I did. I knew I would make it. Throughout this ordeal with Terrence's illness, I learned so much. I learned how strong I was. I was always growing and maintaining a good life for my children. I kept thinking, 'He didn't change me.' Somehow, 'I stayed me!' I appreciated my family, my friends, my teaching job, and my life. I recognized the grief and sadness I experienced, but I somehow managed to stay strong and stand on my own two feet financially at a time when women often didn't even have credit cards. I remember having trouble buying a car on my own, but I was strong, determined, and succeeded. I had so much personal growth and what I call 'integrity with a difference.' It was strengthening, invigorating, and courageous. And I did it with three young children on my own."

**Jocelyn** became a widow at 30 years of age and had two children under the age of 4 years old. She stated, "I think I experienced posttraumatic growth. I grew into a very strong person after my husband's death. I volunteered at my kid's school and in the community. I got to know a lot of people, and people were kind. Finding my way through this traumatic event, this great loss, I grew into someone much stronger than before. My goal was to make our life good and happy. My kid's happiness was always first and foremost. Going through this trauma at age 30 made me look at all the things in my life and triumph as a strong, determined woman."

**Paige**, whose husband died from cancer, reported, "I'm pretty sure I experienced posttraumatic growth. You know the saying, 'What doesn't kill you makes you stronger.' I have been blessed in so many ways. I took the advice that my mother told me years ago: don't make any big decisions for the first year after losing your loved one. I decided to work for a year and not move for a year. I am a business executive who always had a firm grasp on our finances. I would describe myself as strong, but Ben's death made me stronger."

**Maura**, who was in her 20s when her husband, Wesley, was killed in an auto accident, recalled, "It took me a long time to get on with my life from a personal standpoint.

Professionally, I just kept going in my role as a nurse. I threw myself into my work. My work was my life. I forgot about myself, and I lived for my patients, my mother, my sister, and my friends. I closed the door on my married life because it was too painful. I prayed to God for strength, and He gave it to me. I had always been pretty independent, having a career and being well-educated. I had confidence in myself as a professional woman. I had a rewarding career as a nurse and had a master's degree. I was intellectually curious, ambitious, disciplined, and believed in myself to survive. I had a good network of family and friends. I rented an apartment on my own, paid all the bills, got charge accounts in my name, and bought a car on my own for the first time. I surprised myself with my strength and perseverance since I kept my job and didn't move back to my mother's house."

**Cora**, whose husband died waiting for a heart transplant, related, "I had to be strong and simply had to go on because I was left with four boys to raise alone after Brad passed away. You have to just keep going and muster enough strength because they need you, and three of them were still in school. I think Brad's death forced me to grow up. It's easier when there are two parents in the home, and now there was only one. I guess I was stronger than I thought I was. I didn't have a choice; I was the only one there. Somehow, I made it through every day and did what I was supposed to do. I tried to be a good mother, but it is still stressful when you have to do everything alone. I didn't have a lot of help from either of our families because everyone had their problems to deal with and none of us had much money. We lived in government-subsidized housing. I cleaned houses while the kids were in school. You muster up enough strength because there is so much you have to do; at least the kids were not little. I was pretty overwhelmed with life in those days as a widow and having four kids. There was not much time for enjoyment or appreciation of life back then because being a parent took up all of your time. Today, I appreciate my sons and my friends, but life has been hard in general. I have had my share of losses as well as financial stresses. I have had to watch every penny I spend, but I am still thankful. I don't consider myself religious, but I believe in God."

**Marissa**, whose 28-year-old husband died from heat stroke, recounted, "After Rob died, I decided to come back to Rhode Island. All my family was back in Rhode Island. I sold our house, which we had just bought in the New York suburbs, and moved back in with my parents. I eventually bought a house that I had designed and built. One thing that got me through was that I had a strong personality, I was a strong person. I had to be strong for the kids, and I wasn't falling apart mostly for them. I worked a job full-time, I just kept running and kept the household running. After about three years of busy, busy, busy, I slowed down enough to go for counseling and to try to come to terms with Rob's death."

**Lydia** related, "I see myself as a much stronger person now. I guess before Mike died, I didn't give myself much credit. I always followed his lead. Now, I take the lead in my life. I came to learn that I make very good decisions and manage my finances very well."

**Christy**, whose husband died of cancer, remarked, "Being on my own has been a challenge, but I'm a strong person. Nursing and the Army taught me to be a good decision-maker. My husband's death and the loss of his son taught me a greater appreciation for life. I learned to not put off things I wanted to do. My Iraq deployment also taught me that life is short. I prioritize my goals and stick to my plan once I make a plan. It had been quite a while since I was on my own making decisions, but about a year after my husband's death, I put a plan in place and have stuck to it. I am a strong woman who knows my strengths and weaknesses. I am not a 'wallflower' in any respect. I wouldn't have survived in nursing and the Army Reserve for over 30 years if I was a 'wallflower.' I am a leader who attained the rank of colonel in the Army Reserve. I am used to giving orders and accomplishing the mission."

**Marilyn**, whose husband died of a brain tumor at 41, recalled, "I was thrown into a whirlwind, to begin with. I've always been strong, well-informed, and believed in family first. I had my family's support early on and his family's support early on, but as it progressed, we lost some of his family's support because they thought 'We weren't doing enough.' I knew from my background that this was a terminal event and had accepted that, whereas his parents had not accepted that it was a terminal event. They thought he could 'beat' terminal brain cancer. That was a little harder to deal with. You know that you don't want to lose your son before you. I don't think his parents ever accepted that. It was really hard for them to get past that. So, I think that I was their scapegoat. They took a lot of their anxieties out on me. I got connected with a church family, and I don't think I could have made it without them. They gave me the strength to carry on. My church was there helping day by day giving much more support. We did a lot with people from church."

**Barbara's** husband died from his third heart attack at 57 years of age. "I've always been an assertive, strong, accomplished, and successful woman. That did not change after Jack's death. We married when we were in our late 30s, so we were both very established in our careers. In terms of posttraumatic growth, I have grown significantly over the last 15+ years since my husband died. I have matured in so many ways, and I take nothing for granted. I am a financial wizard now and have managed to save money, make good conservative investments, start a Roth IRA, have a good pension from my work, and don't skimp on at least two vacations a year with girlfriends. I maintain my house, have learned to fix toilets and sinks, do mowing and landscaping chores, keep the car in good working order, pay the bills on time, and still find time to read, exercise, care for my dog, and enjoy life."

**Louise**, whose husband died from pancreatic cancer, shared, "I gradually became stronger and more independent after my husband's death. Before, I always let him take the lead in family decisions. It took me about two years to gain my strength, but I was able to become a stronger head of household in many respects. My husband had taught me a lot over the years, and I became a cautious decision-maker. My independence has served me well."

**Patty**, who lost her husband to a stroke after 68 years of marriage, related, "I've always been a strong and capable wife, mother, and woman. Now, at the age of 94, I do water aerobics twice a week, walk two miles every other day with my lady friends, and do weight training at the gym. I have a martini every day at 4 PM."

**Laila**, whose husband died from a cardiac arrhythmia, related, "I'm one tough cookie and always have been one. I just pushed forward. I finished my master's degree after he died. I never took a break, I just kept going. One good friend at work was my biggest cheerleader and mentor. She encouraged me in both my master's program and doctoral program. She would say, 'You can do this. You are a great teacher. You're better than you think you are.' I've been able to move on with my life."

**Joy** stated, "I was determined to have a second healthy baby. It was sheer willpower to try to hang in there for my daughter and this expected baby. Of course, it didn't help that I had nausea and vomiting during the entire pregnancy. Once I came out of my fog because of these tragic events and also not feeling well, I realized that I am a very strong woman. But when you have a young child and are expecting another one, what choice do you have, you have to go on. Family and friends are helpful, but the bottom line is that you have to take care of your child and yourself during the pregnancy. At the time, I was just motivated to keep going for the sake of my daughter and my pregnancy. But you go on for the sake of your children. That's what mothers do."

### Theme: My View of Myself Changed

**Lucinda** recalled, "What changed was that I have discovered that I have the determination not to let negative circumstances rule my life. I have reaffirmed that I am strong, capable, smart, and positive. I did not want to be a bitter woman, and I did not want my children to become bitter about their father's alcoholism. I think in the 1980s, when our marriage ended, it was harder for women to exert their independence, especially financially. Thank God things have changed. I found Al-Anon to be helpful for me and my kids. It showed us that we were not alone. It changed me to better understand my husband's illness and the related problems families of alcoholics face. I became a more open person to let others help me and to not be ashamed about my husband's illness and death." She continued, "I know that my philosophy of life has changed to a certain extent. I believe that we all have new chapters in our lives after traumatic circumstances or a tragedy. I truly believe that now I live in the moment because I don't know what tomorrow will bring. I believe in making things work and asking for help when needed."

**Jocelyn**, whose husband died in his sleep from an undiagnosed cardiac arrhythmia, stated, "I've learned to be a problem solver because I was by myself with two little kids. I've learned to reach out to others when I need help. Over the years I've realized that I'm fine with myself and being alone. I allowed myself to evolve, and I went back to school for my master's degree when my daughter was in college and my son was in high school. I like to teach. I'm a registered nurse, and after my master's degree was completed, I taught licensed practical nurses. When I got my doctorate, I continued to like teaching and have taught at a state college and have been successful. Now, I think my kids are proud of me and view me as a success. I like a challenge, and my work is important to me. I think my philosophy of life has changed somewhat. It's hard to say because I was only 30 when my husband died. I try to keep things on an even keel. I don't have a lot of wants. I'm happy with my house. I'm content with not doing too much at one time. I travel somewhat, but I'd rather be home. My career and my work have become my identity. Being a mother always came first in my life, but now my kids are grown, so work is important to me. I'm a grandmother, and that is very important to me, too."

**Paige** shared, "I felt a change in me after Ben died. I felt different doing ordinary things. I felt different grocery shopping. I felt different on a business trip. I felt like I had nobody to worry about me now. I have to admit that people were wonderful to me. My mother had passed away two years before Ben. I was open to recognizing that my life was changed. My outlook on life did not change because I'm still optimistic and believe in people. I think most people are good, hard-working, kind, and want to do their best."

**Maura** said, "My inner core of being was heartbroken, devastated, and dipped to a level of sadness that I didn't know existed. I felt the loss in my gut as well as in my head and sometimes, I simply felt numb. I felt like my life was ruined and that my dreams were shattered. On a personal level, I was a lost sheep who was having difficulty finding her way but I didn't let anyone know that I felt that way. On the surface, I was strong, determined, and confident because this was my professional demeanor, the one that I let others see.

People kept telling me that I was young and that I'd find love again. I must say that I didn't want to hear those comments, but I think people don't know what to say to a young woman who experiences a great loss. Eventually, I did find love, and it was wonderful. I grew as a person, became even more independent, and realized that I didn't always need to have others around me to be happy and fulfilled. I also had an awareness of my biological clock and prayed that God would give me another chance at love and a family. Fortunately, He came through for me. I surprised myself by opening my heart to someone and getting remarried. We went on to have a family, too. I was able to rebuild my life with my second husband and our two children. For the most part, I filled my life by being attentive to the needs of my husband and children and working full-time when the kids entered preschool. It is only occasionally that I remember my 'battle scars' from my previous loss. When I try to analyze these feelings, I realize that the 'shock' put me in a 'brain fog.' My life felt like a 'bad dream.' Yet, being both a religious and spiritual person, I have always felt that God had a plan for me, and He planned for me to have a family and a successful career. I have always experienced such joy in helping others: family, friends, patients, and co-workers."

**Cora**, whose husband died from heart failure, recalled, "I guess I am stronger than I thought I was. I started to see myself as a strong, independent woman who could provide the essentials for my boys. I learned to live on a very tight budget. With four kids depending on you, you have to stay focused on the job at hand. At the end of the day, I was always very tired. When the boys were in school, I was able to take on a few house-cleaning jobs, which led to extra money. People paid me in cash. My life has been hard, but I have tried to be there for my kids. You have to deal with whatever comes your way. You don't want bad things to happen, but sometimes they do. Some things are not in your control, like my husband's illness."

**Marissa** recalled, "I was always a strong personality who advocated for myself. However, I got even stronger or tougher after Rob's death. For example, when I got a job at the bank, I asked for more money than what they offered. I would not have had the nerve to do that when my husband was alive. I might have thought it, but I would have never come out and said it. This was not the old Marissa; this was the new Marissa. They finally came back to meet my salary demand. I guess I had balls, or they weren't used to dealing with a gutsy or assertive woman."

**Lydia** related, "My life changed, in that some friends disappeared. You hear about a couple of friends disappearing, and that is what happened to me. As a couple, we were very social and used to dance with a polka dance club. After my husband's death, I had nothing in common with this group anymore. I changed, too. I had to force myself to take care of a lot of our finances and the house, things my husband used to do. My car has become my safe zone after my husband died. I can sit in the car and scream and cry and no one hears me but God."

**Christy**, whose husband died of cancer, remarked, "I'm the same person I always was, but have had to learn to do many things alone. Many couples we used to socialize with no longer socialize now that I'm a widow. My family doesn't have frequent contact with me. They never approved of my staying in the Army Reserve, and thought I was crazy to accept the deployments in Germany and especially Iraq. The Army Reserve was part of us and part of our marriage. We met in the Army Reserve, and it was a big piece of what we had in common. We both loved and took pride in being active in the Army Reserve."

**Marilyn**, whose husband died of a brain tumor at 41, said, "I became more accepting of myself and my limitations in raising two boys by myself and being the sole support of our family. I have had to make some forced changes in myself. I became less of a perfectionist and more of a realist. I went from a co-parent to an only parent. My personal growth grew as a result of my situation and experiences. It was more of a forced environment where you had to pick up the pieces of your life. When you have kids, you have to deal with life. You don't have a choice, and you want to do what is best for them. Suck it up and pick up your bootstraps and get going. You're responsible for all the decisions. You are both mother and disciplinarian and father and disciplinarian. That was a real challenge at times, especially with my younger son."

**Barbara's** husband died from his third heart attack at 57 years of age. Barbara related, "My view of myself didn't change very much. I attribute my lack of change to getting married later in life and being well-established in my career before marriage. We did not have any children and were married for a little more than 15 years before Jack's fatal heart attack. The only real change was financial. So, I established a strict budget for myself and stuck to it. I also mourned the loss of many couple friends we had since I was no longer on their social register. To compensate, I reestablished relationships with many of my women friends, and that has worked out very well. I sold our home, built a new house in a less expensive state, and was able to transfer with my company job to the new location."

**Louise**, whose husband died from pancreatic cancer, said, "I was independent to a degree, but always part of a very close couple. He taught me to look on the bright side of everything. I'm like him in terms of outlook; I'm always moving forward. I try to look for the good in people and relationships. I stay positive." She continued, "On another topic, I learned to believe in mediums to hear from the other side. I didn't always believe in that, but a girlfriend took me to a medium and then later to another medium. My husband does visit from the other side. So, I changed by embracing the other side through mediums. I would have never expected this in the 'old' me, but the 'new' me believes in the supernatural and embraces it."

**Patty**, who lost her husband to a stroke after 68 years of marriage, recalled, "I have become more pessimistic about the world because it is hard when you live so long that all of your old friends have passed. I was very content with my life, my marriage, and my four wonderful children. I'm pessimistic because my views on things are changing. I'm not happy, and I'm trying very hard to overcome that attitude. Whether it is politics, the economy, terrorist acts, wars, poverty, and genocide in many countries, the world is changing. I'm 94, and I liked the world much better in the 1950s. It was less complicated, and people were more hopeful and happier then."

**Laila**, whose husband died from a cardiac arrhythmia while taking a nap, related, "I don't think my view of myself has changed. I always try to be confident in situations. But sometimes I question myself. I think it is normal and natural to question yourself. I believe that your life experiences make up who you are and how you act. You have a different type of knowledge base because of your life experiences. I am hard on myself at times, and overly critical. You know, 'shoulda, woulda, coulda,' I have done that all my life. Yet, perseverance has been a key characteristic in my life. I push through and hang in there. I try to set a good example and be a good role model and a mentor for others. I still believe in the same values and strive to do a good job in all that I do. I am fair and honest. I try to be helpful and hardworking."

Table 3.1 Widowed Women Demographics

| Name | Age at Interview | Cause of Husband's Death | Woman's Occupation | Reported Socioeconomic Status |
|---|---|---|---|---|
| Lucinda | 61 | Chronic alcoholism | Elementary teacher | Middle |
| Cora | 62 | Heart failure | House cleaner | Lower |
| Lydia | 64 | Pancreatic cancer | Secretary | Middle |
| Marilyn | 58 | Brain tumor | School nurse | Middle |
| Christy | 54 | Cancer | Nurse | Middle |
| Paige | 57 | Melanoma | Financial officer | Upper |
| Barbara | 68 | Heart failure | Teacher | Middle |
| Louise | 62 | Pancreatic cancer | Real estate agent | Middle |
| Patty | 94 | Stroke | Retired | Middle |
| Clarice | 57 | Cardiac arrest | Bank teller | Middle |
| Jocelyn | 45 | Cardiac arrest | Nurse | Middle |
| Maura | 33 | Car accident | Graduate student | Middle |
| Marisa | 38 | Heat stroke | Bank manager | Middle |
| Laila | 63 | Heart attack | Professor | Middle |
| Joy | 64 | Heart attack | Teacher | Middle |

The aforementioned narratives present changes in a widow's life after losing her husband or partner to death through the lens of PTG. Although each widow's journey was different, as was her relationship with her partner before this loss, most of these women experienced some degree of PTG in the time since the loss. Many were surprised by the advances and trajectories their journey encompassed. There is no set path for their journeys since achieving some degree of PTG is individualized and enhanced by many unique factors such as personality, social support, family relationships, compassion for themselves and others, and the ability to vacate one's comfort zone to embrace new possibilities or opportunities.

## References

Asai, M., Matsui, Y., & Uchitomi, Y. (2013). Patterns of coping strategies after bereavement among spouses of cancer patients. *Shinrigaku Kenkyu, 84*(5), 498–507. https://doi.org/10.4992/jjpsy.84.498

Bennett, K. M., Gibbons, K., & Mackensie-Smith, S. (2010). Loss and restoration in later life: An examination of the dual process method of coping with bereavement. *Omega—Journal of Death and Dying, 61*(4), 315–322. https://doi.org/10.2190/OM.61.4.d

Bennett, K. M., & Soulsby, L. K. (2012). Well-being in bereavement and widowhood. *Illness, Crisis and Loss, 20*(4), 321–337. https://doi.org/10.2190/IL.20.4.b

Das, A. (2013). Spousal loss and health in late life: moving beyond emotional trauma. *Journal of Aging and Health, 25*(2), 221–242.

DiGiacomo, M., Davidson, P. M., Byles, J., & Nolan, M. (2013). An integrative and socio-cultural perspective of health, wealth, and adjustment in widowhood. *Health Care Women International, 34*(12), 1067–1083. https://doi.org/10.1080/07399332.2012.712171

DiGiacomo, M., Lewis, J., Nolan, M., Phillips, J., & Davidson, P. (2013a). Health transitions in recently widowed older women: A mixed methods study. *BMC Health Services Research, 13*(143), 37–47.

DiGiacomo, M., Lewis, J., Nolan, M., Phillips, J., & Davidson, P. (2013b). Transitioning from caregiving to widowhood. *Journal of Pain and Symptom Management, 46*, 817–825.

DiGiacomo, M., Lewis, J., Phillips, J., Nolan, M., & Davidson, P. M. (2015). The business of death: A qualitative study of financial concerns of widowed older women. *BMC Women's Health, 15*, 36–44. https://doi.org/10.1186/s12905-015-0194-1

Doherty, M. E., & Scannell-Desch, E. A. (2021). Posttraumatic growth in women who have experienced the loss of their spouse or partner. *Nursing Forum, 51*(9), 1–9. https://doi.org/10.1111/nuf.12657

Eshbaugh, E. (2008). Perceptions of living alone among older adult women. *Journal of Community Health Nursing, 25*, 125–137.

Guldin, M. B., Jensen, A. B., Zachariae, R., & Vedsted, P. (2013). Healthcare utilization of bereaved relatives of patients who died from cancer. A national population-based study. *Psychooncology, 22*(5), 1152–1158.

Hansford, M., & Jobson, L. (2021). Associations between relationship quality, social network resources, appraisals, coping, and posttraumatic stress disorder symptoms. *Psychological Trauma: Theory, Research, Practice, and Policy, 13*(5), 575–585. https://doi.org/10.1037/tra0001015

Kenen, R. (2021). Uncoupled: American widows in times of uncertainty and ambiguous norms. *Journal of Contemporary Ethnography, 50*, 1–30. https://doi.org/10:1177/08912416200801

King, B. M., Carr, D. C., & Taylor, M. G. (2019). Depressive symptoms and the buffering effect of resilience on widowhood by gender. *The Gerontologist, 59*(6), 1122–1130. https://doi.org/10.1093/geront/gny115

Kristiansen, C. B., Kjær, J. N., Hjorth, P., Andersen, K., & Prina, A. M. (2019a). Prevalence of common mental disorders in widowhood: A systematic review and meta-analysis. *Journal of Affective Disorders, 15245*, 1016–1023. https://doi.org/10.1016/j.jad.2018.11.088

Kristiansen, C. B., Kjaer, J. N., Hjorth, P., Andersen, K., & Prina, A. M. (2019b). The association of time since spousal loss and depression in widowhood: A systematic review and meta-analysis. *Social Psychiatry and Psychiatric Epidemiology, 54*(7), 781–792. https://doi.org/10.1007/s00127-019-01680-3

Lancaster, H., & Johnson, T. (2020). Losing a partner: The varying financial and practical impacts of bereavement in different sociodemographic groups. *British Medical Journal of Supportive & Palliative Care, 33*(7), 37–46. https://doi.org/10:e17

Mark, K., Stevelink, S., Choi, J., & Fear, N. (2018). Posttraumatic growth in the military: A systematic review. *Occupational and Environmental Medicine, 75*(12), 904–915.

Moon, J. R., Kondo, N., Glymour, M. M., & Subramanian, S. V. (2011). Widowhood and mortality: A meta-analysis. *PloS One, 6*(8), e23465. https://doi.org/10.1371/journal.pone.0023465

Mostofsky, M., Maclure, M., Sherwood, J. B., Tofler, G. H., Muller, J. E., & Mittleman, M. A. (2012). Risk of acute myocardial infarction after death of a significant person in one's life. *Circulation, 125*(3), 491–496. https://doi.org/10.1161/CIRCULATIONAHA.111.061770

Ramadas, S., & Kuttichira, P. (2013). Bereavement leading to death. *Asian Journal of Psychiatry, 6*(2), 184–185. https://doi.org/10.1016/j.ajp.2012.09.002

Roberts, A. R., & Adams, K. B. (2018). Quality of life trajectories of older adults living in senior housing. *Research on Aging, 11*(8), 26–34. https://doi.org/10.1177/0164027517713313

Scannell-Desch, E. A. (2005a). Mid-life widows narratives of support and non-support. *Journal of Psychosocial Nursing, 43*(4), 39–47.

Scannell-Desch, E. A. (2005b). Struggles and triumphs of middle-aged widows. *Journal of Hospice and Palliative Nursing Care, 23*(1), 17–22.

Stroebe, M., Schut, H., & Stroebe, W. (2007). Health outcomes of bereavement. *Lancet, 370*(9603), 1960–1967.

# 4

# POSTTRAUMATIC GROWTH IN WOMEN WHO HAVE EXPERIENCED THE LOSS OF A CHILD

The loss of a child is one of the most devastating and horrific experiences a parent can ever endure. Bereaved parents are forced to deal with core questions of human existence. They have to face the disruption of what is perceived to be the natural course of life, with children outliving their parents. The impact of losing a child of any age can persist for years (Riley et al., 2007; Worden, 2008). Several researchers have reported that grief and sorrow from losing a child tend to be more intense, disruptive, and longer-lasting than other kinds of losses, particularly for mothers (Keesee et al., 2008; Worden, 2008). Healthcare providers need to understand the factors that help mothers cope effectively with their loss to prevent maladaptive behaviors and promote posttraumatic growth (Baskin & Enright, 2004; Enright & Fitzgibbons, 2014; Wade et al., 2014).

**What Does the Research Tell Us?**

Mothers grieve the loss of their child in a variety of ways based on their culture, personality, spirituality, core beliefs, and the mix of attributes that make them individual and unique people. It is an intricate complex of emotional, behavioral, cognitive, and physiological reactions after the loss of a loved one (Worden, 2008). Anger appears to be a significant element of grief over the loss of a child (Cook et al., 2002; Ronel & Lebel, 2006; Saka & Cohen-Louck, 2014). Parents often express anger at themselves, hospitals, healthcare providers, family, friends, and God.

Attempts to decrease feelings of anger and restore well-being in bereaved mothers may prove to be quite challenging and difficult to achieve (Cook et al., 2002). Mental health providers use many psychological approaches and techniques in grief counseling and therapy. Some of these therapeutic modalities include forgiveness therapy (Enright & Fitzgibbons, 2014), interpersonal therapy (Crenshaw, 2006), and meaning-oriented therapy (Neimeyer et al., 2010; Neimeyer et al., 2014; Neimeyer, 2016). Experts in the field of grief counseling have not reached a consensus on the most efficacious approach because grief following loss is individual. It cannot be addressed by a 'one-size-fits-all' perspective.

DOI: 10.4324/9781003456650-4

Martincekova and Klatt (2017) in their work on grief, forgiveness, and posttraumatic growth emphasize the need for more research on interventions to decrease grief in mothers. Their sample consisted of 60 grieving mothers from Slovakia who completed three grief inventories. The results showed a negative association between forgiveness and grief and a strong positive association between forgiveness and PTG.

The notion of PTG has been applied to bereavement and grief research (Calhoun et al., 2010). Michael and Cooper (2013) conducted a systematic review of PTG, which demonstrated that PTG can certainly be experienced by bereaved individuals. These researchers were careful to emphasize that growth does not mean that distress ceases. They point out that both experiences can occur at the same time, which agrees with the seminal work of Tedeschi and Calhoun (1995, 1996, 2004). Michael and Cooper (2013) identified potential mediators for the emergence of growth such as social support, time since death, religion or spirituality, and active coping strategies. Their systematic review addressed questions concerning specific aspects of PTG and factors that could facilitate PTG or prevent PTG.

Many researchers reported parents' experiences of positive growth as well as parents' ongoing sadness. Growth and sadness can be experienced like a seesaw going up and down or a roller-coaster or waves going out and then coming in on a beach. This illustrates the paradox of PTG. In a study by Reilly and colleagues (2008), participants reported many grief symptoms, including anger and despair after their child's death. However, they also mentioned that their grief became easier to manage over time.

Buchi and colleagues (2007) highlighted that 80% of parents show signs of grief two to six years after their premature baby died. Gerrish and associates (2014) found that despite mothers being able to see personal strength in themselves, they also acknowledged continued sadness. Similarly, other researchers mentioned that bereaved parents often have long-term psychological responses after loss such as increased depression (Rogers et al., 2008), anxiety (Buchi et al., 2007), and complicated grief (Zetumer et al., 2015). They were also found to have relationship difficulties after losing a child (Rogers et al., 2008) and poorer physical health (Li et al., 2002). Even if the child is a grown adult at the time of death, parents are likely to view the death as unnatural and untimely because they are faced with the difficult task of trying to find some way to continue life without their child (Wheeler, 2002).

PTG proposes that in the struggle to cope with trauma and in addition to experiencing negative symptoms, positive personal changes are possible. Along this same line of thinking, three studies described the experience of intense grief as an important factor in the development of PTG. Buchi and colleagues (2007) found a positive association between grief and growth scores when anxiety and depression scores were controlled. Engelkemeyer and Marwit (2008) in a multiple regression analysis found that grief intensity accounted for only 4% of the variance of PTG scores in their study. Gerrish and associates (2014) reported that women who experienced high, but not overwhelming, levels of grief experienced more growth in the long run.

It is important to note that many quantitative and mixed methods studies use the Posttraumatic Growth Inventory (PTGI) to measure PTG. The PTGI (Tedeschi & Calhoun, 1996) is a 21-item Likert scale designed to assess PTG across the five PTG domains: new possibilities, relating to others, personal growth, spiritual change, and appreciation of life. The inventory has demonstrated good validity and reliability (Tedeschi & Calhoun, 1996). For example, Jenewein and collagues (2008) conducted a study that involved parents of premature infants and found that bereaved parents had higher PTGI scores overall when compared to the PTGI scores of parents whose premature babies had survived.

When we examine research that reflected the various domains of Tedeschi and Calhoun's PTG model (1995), a host of qualitative, quantitative, and mixed methods studies surfaced. Bogensperger and Lueger-Schuster's (2014) study aimed to expand on existing work about meaning reconstruction in a sample of bereaved parents. These researchers emphasized that this type of loss caused the parents to ponder core questions of human existence (Currier et al., 2010; Keesee et al., 2008). Bereaved parents must deal with the rupture of a widely shared concept of what is perceived to be the natural course of events in life, that parents precede their children in death. Specifically, the researchers examined the relationship between meaning reconstruction, complicated grief, and PTG with particular attention to unexpected and traumatic deaths.

According to Bogensperger and Lueger-Schuster (2014), the process of finding and integrating the meaning of the loss and its aftermath into one's worldview occurs. Sense-making refers to thinking processes to understand the loss by incorporating it into a personal worldview. Benefit-finding refers to discovering positive consequences in the face of adversity. For example, increased empathy or compassion for others would be viewed as a benefit. Therefore, changes in one's identity in the aftermath of tragedy can be viewed as PTG (Tedeschi & Calhoun, 1996).

In the Bogensperger and Lueger-Schuster (2014) study, personal growth themes were more commonly identified with participants reporting "being more tolerant" and "developing personal potential." One-third of participants described a desire to help others, especially other bereaved parents. Participants also reported having a reduced focus on work and financial issues and an increased focus on family life. One of the least mentioned themes or domains in this study was an appreciation of life. Yet, 11 of the 30 participants reported having a heightened appreciation of "living in the moment" and not taking things for granted. These researchers noted that participants in their study did not discuss the death of their child in terms of it being "God's will." They suggested that referring to God might reflect the prevalence of religion in America compared to European countries. They reported a positive relationship between meaning reconstruction and PTG. They identified 20 sense-making themes in their study and specified that the most common theme was the purpose of the child's life and death.

Existential growth refers to changes in how living in the world is perceived and understood. This includes the meaning of life, spirituality, and religious views. In the Brabant et al. (1997) study, all participants mentioned a fundamental change in themselves after the loss of a child. Many considered themselves more sensitive and realized how precious life is. Some placed a greater emphasis on religion and felt more spiritual than they did before the death. They mentioned that prayers and rituals were an important resource. Several commented that "finding God" and "being more spiritual" helped them. Ten participants reported an increased desire to help others. However, if the child died by suicide, the parents did not score highly on the domain of new possibilities on the PTGI (18%) compared to the other four domains. One parent in this study described themselves as a "failure." Brabant and colleagues (1997) suggested that this might be because this participant had the shortest amount of time between the death and participation in the study.

Buchi and associates (2007) shared that participants in their study had the highest scoring on the PTGI for "stronger than I thought I was" and "knowing I can handle difficulties." While the bereaved mothers in their study had higher grief scores, they also had higher growth scores. They also reported having increased compassion for others and indicated that they knew they could "count on people in times of trouble." Buchi and associates (2007) documented that 78% of bereaved mothers and 44% of bereaved fathers reported that they discovered new possibilities related to "what is important in life" since the death of their baby.

Buchi and associates (2007) emphasized that healthcare providers should be aware of the potential for long-lasting positive and negative changes after the death of a child. For example, if parents have a very limited support network this could put them at greater risk following the death of a child. Foot and colleagues (2014) recognized the value of putting newly bereaved parents in touch with previously bereaved parents to encourage the development of "expert-by-experience" services. Similarly, Calhoun and colleagues (2010) discuss a model of working with bereaved individuals called "expert companionship" to facilitate PTG. These interventions are a clinical approach that includes respect, sensitivity to wavering emotions, and appreciation of the paradox of PTG. Researchers need to be cautious in analyzing the changes that occur in parents' lives after the loss of a child and not assume PTG or PTSD.

In a study by Gerrish and associates (2014), meaning-making phenomena underlying the responses of 13 bereaved mothers who lost their children to cancer were investigated. All mothers reported having continuing bonds with their children. They mentioned visiting the cemetery and speaking aloud to their child. They emphasized the importance of maintaining relationships and doing community work, such as cancer awareness. This drew on the legacy of the child which facilitated PTG. The mothers focused on their continued love for their children and how they treasured mementos such as photos, favorite toys, games, and books. Some participants took the perspective that their child would want them to enjoy life again. They described how showing compassion and support for others helped them with their healing and fostered their transformation. They believed that the social environment had the potential to further their PTG, especially when they could tell their story and share their feelings with a non-judgmental listener.

Gerrish and colleagues (2014) commented that having other children may have served a protective function for mothers. Having the responsibility of other children to raise may have distracted a woman to a certain extent, keeping her from completely focusing on the child she lost to death. Findings identified specific characteristics, coping processes, and factors to distinguish adaptive as opposed to complicated grief responses after this type of loss. Mothers' assumptions about themselves, other people, and their world appeared to facilitate meaningful changes in their self-identify. These changes surfaced after they struggled with trauma and grief, and they often led to personal growth. The mothers acquired a more flexible view of major life events and greater integration of the loss into the narrative about themselves. Additionally, they were able to give a more adaptive evaluation of themselves at the time of the child's death. Thus, the loss reinforced and strengthened elements of their pre-loss self-identity. Conversely, some mothers showed problematic changes to their self-identities after the loss. Complicated grief responses were thought to be a product of maladaptive processes and might have reaffirmed certain negative behaviors held by the mothers before their loss (Gerrish et al., 2014).

A major way that the 13 women found solace in their loss was to establish a special and symbolic bond with their deceased child. Adaptation appeared to be slightly easier when the mother had time to prepare and anticipate the death of her child. The cancer diagnosis and poor prognosis helped most mothers face the reality of the situation. This was not to imply that all hope was lost. All 13 bereaved mothers reported that they continued to have a permanent feeling of sadness and that they expected this would be a life-long feeling (Gerrish et al., 2014).

Moore and colleagues (2015) suggested that participants' scores of growth in their study were lower than expected. They believe that this may have been because their study included bereaved parents who lost a child within the previous two years. The two-year time period may have been a barrier in measuring growth. These participants most strongly endorsed the "relating to others" subscale of the PTGI (Tedeschi & Calhoun, 1996). Moore and associates (2015) reported that participants indicated an increased appreciation for life on the PTGI (33%) and a spiritual change (34%). These researchers documented that participants who told of new possibilities possessed the personality traits of openness to experience, neuroticism, and resilience. Similarly, more personal growth was linked to active coping and support-seeking behaviors.

Reilly and colleagues (2008) reported that mothers whose children died more recently had greater difficulty identifying growth. These researchers found that some of the mothers who perceived a positive experience attributed this to their relief that their child was no longer suffering from a terminal illness. The participants shared that they benefitted from being with other bereaved mothers because they felt that these other mothers were the only people who truly understood what they had experienced. All mothers in this study shared that they were involved with charities or social service agencies and their mission was to use their traumatic experience to support others and that it benefitted them personally. A character trait or quality that helped to predict PTG in mothers was optimism (Helgeson et al., 2006; Reilly et al., 2008). Some mothers reported occasionally masking their emotions when it did not feel appropriate to talk about their child, despite wanting to.

It is important to note that Reilly and colleagues' (2008) study was not done in the United States. It reported that women who already had religion in their lives questioned their beliefs but did not change them. Conversely, women in the study who did not have religious faith before the death of their child did not turn to religion when their child died.

A study by Jenewein and others (2008) noted that mothers expressed more PTG than fathers. This was evident in the PTGI subscale "relating to others" with mothers scoring significantly higher in this domain than any other domain. Some mothers felt that they were coping with the loss differently than their husbands. This made emotion-focused activities such as looking at photos more difficult.

It is noteworthy to mention that PTG is a relatively recent area of empirical study (Tedeschi & Calhoun, 1995) and that conducting a research study with bereaved parents is a sensitive area. The findings of the studies discussed in this literature review indicate that bereaved parents were able to experience elements of PTG such as changes in self-identity, increased positive relationships, appreciation of life, changes in priorities, and changes in spirituality. The time interval since the child's death and agreeing to participate in a research study appeared to be an important consideration associated with PTG. It was suggested by several researchers that a longer time interval since the death allowed parents a chance to experience more elements of PTG (Helgeson et al., 2006). Research suggests that there are multiple factors associated with fostering or impeding PTG. Such factors include cognitive processes, social networks, other bereaved families, continuing bonds, sense-making, and personal characteristics (Waugh et al., 2018).

The literature supports the seminal research of Tedeschi and Calhoun (1995) that individuals need to experience distress and struggle to realize PTG. Two recent systematic reviews helped identify and discuss PTG in bereaved populations (Michael & Cooper, 2013; Waugh et al., 2018). These two systematic reviews were congruent with the meta-analysis of Helgeson and coworkers (2006), which reported that women usually perceive more benefits from a traumatic event related to their coping strategies.

A powerful insight mentioned in this literature review highlights the importance of having bereaved parents interact with parents who had previously endured the loss of a child. It is of paramount importance for newly bereaved parents to know they are not alone. While some people have strong support systems with abundant family and friends, others may not be blessed with the quantity or quality. It is also important to recognize that participants in the aforementioned studies were volunteers. The same is true about the four qualitative studies conducted by the authors of this book. Most people choose to participate to help others and to advance science, specifically the healthcare professions, and psychology. Participants detailing their experiences of losing a child to death are usually recruited from support groups or in the case of this book from a broad nursing network of colleagues from universities, hospitals, and professional organizations who have access to numerous people who met the study's inclusion criteria.

The studies mentioned in this literature review should be viewed in the context of their limitations and focus particularly on the varied and unique experiences of bereaved parents. It is their "lived experience" that the reader should appreciate and remember. Every study participant will vary in terms of prior mental well-being, social support, and potential for PTG. Although there are indications of growth and possible ways to enhance its development, the findings cannot be generalized. Future research is needed, especially in the qualitative arena, to gain a greater understanding of PTG. Longitudinal and mixed methods research with larger and more diverse samples would also add to knowledge development on this topic.

### Our Study Themes

The following themes emerged from the current study conducted by the researchers/authors. The themes are listed to guide the reader in delving into the stories of nine mothers and two grandmothers who lived through the experience of loss. The themes were formulated after data analysis, and it is hoped that they will guide the reader to understand and appreciate the stories. These themes are (1) unanticipated and anticipated loss; (2) when I lost my child, I lost part of myself; (3) picking up the pieces of my life; (4) support, kindness, and compassion helped; (5) moving on while still broken; (6) never forgotten, always in my heart; and (7) holding my loved ones close.

### Our Study Methods

As with our previously cited study we conducted with widows, our study on the loss of a child employed purposive and snowball sampling. It is important to note that the two grandmothers who participated in this study were nurses who were closely involved with the newborn's care and were of great support to the parents. Both grandmothers heard about the study and asked to participate. Study participants were recruited through the investigators' nursing network, which comprised faculty and clinical colleagues at affiliated hospitals. Institutional Review Board approval was granted by the university where the first author was employed. Inclusion criteria were women who identified themselves as a mother or grandmother who lost a child through death; the ability to read, write, and speak English; the ability to recall the experience of the child's death; and willingness to discuss the experience. We decided that a minimal five-year period between the death and research interview was a reasonable interval to allow for adjustment. Yet, most time intervals were substantially longer. Potential participants who met inclusion criteria were mailed a letter explaining the study and the concept of PTG. A consent form and return mailing envelope were included for those interested in participating in the study. Eleven consent forms and demographic information sheets were completed and returned. After written consent was obtained, an email was sent to schedule an interview at the participant's convenience. Data were collected from Fall 2020 through Fall 2021. A mental health nurse practitioner was available for debriefing if any participant became upset or felt uncomfortable during or after the interview. None of the participants needed debriefing or counseling.

## Theme: Unanticipated and Anticipated Loss

When death was expected because of a serious illness, there was time to prepare for the inevitable even though it was difficult, sad, and heartbreaking. Anticipation allowed for some preparation and coming to terms with the trajectory of the serious health issue. However, when death was sudden and unexpected, it came without warning and put loved ones in a state of shock and disbelief. The following quotes illustrate both unanticipated and anticipated loss.

### Unanticipated Loss

**Mother**: Amanda
**Child**: Carol

"My 3-year-old daughter had been diagnosed with Crohn's disease about a year and a half before she died but that was not the reason for her death. She developed a gastric volvulus. She was three, and I was working doing private duty. I remember one time, several months before she died, Joe called me and said that Carol says she's in a lot of pain in her stomach and I'm not sure what to do for her. We didn't think anything of it, and it kind of spontaneously resolved. What do you do with something that spontaneously resolves? We didn't think further about it. Now, months later, we had been to a 'Disney on Ice' show on Saturday afternoon and we stopped at McDonald's for dinner on the way home. That night Carol started feeling sick to her stomach, and she was up several times vomiting, but it was in small amounts. I did call the pediatrician, and he didn't think too much of it because it was December and lots of kids had gastrointestinal viruses. It might have had to do with McDonald's and that's probably what he thought, too. He said he was getting a lot of calls about kids that were having a virus where they were vomiting so it didn't sound like anything out of the ordinary. So, Carol was up on and off during the night, but she did get some sleep. So, Joe and I decided that he would sleep upstairs.

Our bedroom was on the first floor, so Carol slept in the bed with me. She was up and down all night vomiting, but it was just small amounts. I didn't think anything was all that wrong because she wasn't acting hideously sick. At about 7:00 AM, Joe came down, but Carol still didn't seem overtly ill, but the vomiting was continuing. So, I decided to go get some sleep upstairs with Joe keeping an eye on Carol because she was still vomiting. I was asleep for maybe an hour or two, and Joe came upstairs and told me that Carol's abdomen was swollen and that he wanted me to look at it. I came downstairs and looked at her, and her abdomen was completely distended, and I knew something was very wrong. I called the doctor's office and left a message with the answering service for the pediatrician that we were on our way to the emergency room. We didn't know what was wrong with her. We got her to the emergency room between 9:00 AM and 9:30 AM that Sunday morning. We had called Joe's parents who live nearby to pick up Scott because he was six years old and had traveled with us to the emergency room. Joe's parents met us at the emergency room and took Scott back to their house. The ER people took Carol in, and she was still responding and talking to us. I remember they tried to get a blood pressure reading on her and couldn't get one. They tried different blood pressure cuffs from the pediatric unit. But Carol was talking to us and saying that she was hungry. We finally realized that things were really serious by this time. Our pediatrician said he'd like to call in a critical care specialist who was another doctor who had been in the practice with him but had left the practice to become a pediatric critical care specialist. Everyone in the ER was working on Carol. The whole sight worried me as a nurse; it spelled things to me that Carol was crashing! They said to us, 'Is there anybody that you want to call? I said, 'I want to call my sister, Kate,' so I called her and told her that I was not sure what was going on, but that Carol was in really bad shape. My sister was almost two hours away, and she is also a nurse, and she said, 'I'm coming down.' Her kids were young, so she left the kids with my mother and told my mother, 'You better start praying.' My sister remembers that it was the most beautiful day, it was clear, and the sky was blue. She said that she wondered, 'What the heck am I going to find out when I get to the hospital.' We asked the unit secretary in the ER to call our church. She had to leave a message on the answering machine probably because it was Sunday morning, and the priest was saying Mass. The priest showed up shortly to see what was going on. My father-in-law came over, too. At around 11:00 AM, the doctor said, 'We think she has toxic megacolon. She's in bad shape.' A Code Blue was called, and I remember thinking that something must have happened to someone on the team working on Carol. How ridiculous of me to think that, and not think that it was Carol. They took her to the operating room still doing chest compressions. They had called in an on-call general surgeon. I later thought, 'That poor guy getting stuck with this mess.' They told us the surgery was going to take a couple of hours. We were in the waiting room with my father-in-law, the priest, and a nursing supervisor who was nice and stuck with us. I didn't realize how horrible the situation was. Well, I don't think we were in the waiting room more than 20 or 30 minutes when the surgeon came out and said, 'We couldn't save her.' I remember screaming. 'Oh my God, my baby.' Another person waiting in the ER waiting room got up and ran out because she didn't want to hear it. My father-in-law was with us, and our pastor was with us so we had support. The whole experience was just so unbelievable. I think they put the time of death as 12:05 PM. In a little more than three hours, she was gone. My father-in-law was beside himself. I told him not to tell Scott. Joe and I wanted to tell Scott that Carol had died. The surgeon explained to us that Carol's stomach was twisted at both ends and that's why she was vomiting such small amounts. Her stomach had ruptured."

"My sister said when she walked into the ER, she knew something bad had happened because when she gave them our names, they said we'll take you right up to the OR. Keep in mind this was 1987, so there were no cell phones. My sister was driving down without any way to communicate. To be honest, it's interesting to recall what I remember from that horrible day. We had the car seat in the car and just looking at it made Joe whip it out of the car and throw it in the trunk. We wouldn't need it anymore. I remember my mother-in-law telling me not to cry in front of Scott. I thought, 'How could I not cry?'"

"I didn't even have time to process this whole experience, but I had to notify people. I called my friend Jean who just a few days before had a D&C following a miscarriage. She was a mess, and I remember almost exactly what I said to her. She and I had daughters three days apart but now mine was gone. Jean was a nurse, too, and we had gone through graduate school together. They moved to Ohio some years later, but we're still friends, so then I asked her to call my college friend, Peggy. Peggy then called everyone in our large circle of friends. I mean Peggy was the one that did all the work. She called everybody because I certainly wasn't capable of it."

"I thought my kid had a stomach virus. I felt so incredibly guilty that I was so stupid that I didn't recognize that it was something very serious. I felt so guilty about the whole thing. Until Joe said that Carol's abdomen was distended, I didn't think it was anything out of the ordinary. We had her wake on Tuesday night and the funeral on Wednesday. People were so good to us, the doorbell kept ringing as people dropped off stuff. People dropped food and people sent flowers and other things, I mean it was just non-stop. Peggy moved into my house and ran my house for me for the next couple of days."

"This is silly, but this is how I felt every time the doorbell rang, I kept thinking that the police would be coming to arrest me. I felt like the people in the emergency room must have reported me to the police because nobody could be that stupid. They're coming to arrest me. I'm thinking that someone felt that this 'moron mother' should be arrested. Well, we all beat ourselves up and think that as nurses we are supposed to save the world. With Crohn's disease, Carol was on different medications, and we were so compliant with her treatment plan. We'd even wake her up if she was due for medication. It never occurred to me that things would get out of hand as massively as they did."

"I went to see the surgeon who operated on Carol a couple of weeks later and my sister went with me, and he said, 'I've never seen anything like that,' and he said he did some research because he said it is 'so rare.' It was bizarre, so as it turned out she didn't have a lot of what is called the omentum. It's supposed to hold your organs tightly in place in the abdomen. So that's why her stomach was able to move around so much. Crohn's disease appears to do with the omentum problem. It was like there was something wrong with her gastrointestinal tract really from the beginning. There were a few other odd things like the way her teeth came in, and one of her kidneys was not quite in the right position. But all the tests came back negative. I guess weird stuff was going on with her related to the gastrointestinal tract, but you know, there was no way to put it together and there were no real red flags."

**Amanda** continued, "After Carol died, I think I went to full-time at the community hospital. I also joined Compassionate Friends, which is a support group for bereaved parents, and I went to the first meeting a month after Carol died, and I went pretty much every month for a couple of years. At one of those meetings, I met a woman who had lost her adult daughter.

The daughter was 38 when she died, and the woman was in her 60s. We became very good friends, and after a couple of years, we became the co-leaders of a Compassionate Friends group. We were able to help the newly bereaved. I think with Compassionate Friends, we did it for two years, and then we said was time for somebody else to pass it on to. I went to some conferences, and I do feel that it helped me. I also feel like I was able to help other parents who had lost children, even adult children. It just seemed to work for me. Joe wanted nothing to do with Compassion Friends. He said it made him even sadder to hear other people's stories. He did go a little bit in the beginning. The other thing that happened when I was at the community hospital a couple of times, maybe three at the most, there would be someone coming into the ER, and it would be a child that died, and somebody knew about my experience and they asked me to go down and talk to the parents. I wanted to turn around and help someone because of my experience. I realized that people listen to you more when you have been through a similar experience. It gives you credibility. People realize that you understand their situation intimately."

**Amanda** added, "I had great support from my sister. My sister called me every single night. Now, this was back when you had to pay for long-distance calls, and she was going through a divorce from her husband and working probably three jobs. She called me every single night for months and months and months and so did Peggy. I would talk to them every night, and I would tell the same story over and over again and they never said anything; they just let me ramble on aimlessly. I had a lot of support there. Then, I did private duty for two basic patients. One was a man who had Parkinson's disease, and his home was only five minutes from here. Then, the other was a lady who had been at home and was now in a nursing home. The people at the agency who worked on both cases were just wonderful to me. They told me to arrange my schedule to fit in with being there for my son. With one family, they let me pick up Scott from school and bring him there for milk and cookies. People were wonderful to me. I felt like I had a wonderful support system."

"Joe and I talked about things from the beginning, and we knew that the chance of a marriage making it after losing a child was very low. There is a 90% divorce rate. We knew that we had to work on our marriage. Also, we had a six-year-old son. From the Compassionate Friends group I attended, I saw marriages that were breaking up, and I also saw other ones that were growing stronger together. I'm sure having another child is an impetus to try to make it work if you want to have a normal life."

"I remember Joe's parents were a little surprised that we were going to have a wake and funeral. I went over to the funeral home the afternoon of the wake, and the funeral director was wonderful. He asked me if I had any other children. I said, 'Yes, we have a six-year-old,' and he said that 'Kids are more scared of what they don't know than what they do know,' and he said, 'If you think you can do it, I would recommend that you bring your son over to see Carol.' Joe said that he just couldn't do it again. My mother was staying at my house, and she was the strongest person you could ever imagine. So, we brought Scott over and Carol looked very peaceful, like she was just sleeping. She didn't look like she was in pain, and she didn't look scary. She was dressed in her Christmas dress, and I felt like this was the right thing to do for Scott."

"The summer before Carol died, we went to Disney World, and I remember having fun memories. We had a wonderful time at Disney World and have nice pictures and I think that sort of makes me glad that we went. Joe wanted to wait till the kids were older. But, with everything that happened, we were glad for the memories."

**Amanda** stated, "As a nurse, I have always considered myself a very compassionate person. After going through this traumatic, sad, and horrendous experience, I have put myself out there to help others even more. Having lost a child myself, people listened to me and could relate to me. I had credibility with them. Helping others also helped me. Before losing Carol, I used to think I was a wimp. Eventually, I realized how strong I am. It surprised me at first. I feel like I have a reasonably healthy life going forward."

**Amanda** added, "I believe in not putting things off. I am so glad we took the trip to Disney World when Carol was turning three years old, and Scott was six years old. It gave us special family memories before Carol's sudden death. I believe in enjoying things as they happen and making the most of life. Family and friends are so important."

**Mother**: Susan
**Child**: Brianne

"We were so shocked when we got the call. Our daughter, Brianne, took a bottle of pills after a break-up with her boyfriend at college. They had been having relationship problems, and after he ended it, Brianne was angry, depressed, and heartbroken and decided to end her life. She was a bright and beautiful girl, an A student, and had everything going for her. This act was unlike anything she had ever done before. I'm sure she did it in a fit of anger. She didn't contact anyone; she just did it. She left a note saying that she didn't want to live without Jason and that she saw no way out of her broken heart. It was so awful, and there was nothing we could do; she was gone. We were numb, and we had to drive to the college immediately. We left our younger children with relatives. Brianne was our oldest child. We were horrified, devastated, and could not believe the situation. My husband and I went over and over things, talking about Brianne, as we drove to the college. It was at least a six-hour drive, and we were all talked out by the time we arrived. We had never experienced anything so painful and profoundly sad in our lives."

**Susan** continued, "It was a shocking and painful experience for our family. Eventually, we had to come to terms with Brianne's death. I was numb for a long time and in disbelief. I also felt guilty that Brianne didn't call me and talk to me about her feelings because maybe I could have helped her or gotten some help for her."

**Mother**: Penny
**Child**: Joseph

"The loss of my son, Joseph, was a bitterly painful experience. It was so unexpected. He was scuba diving and I guess had some type of heart failure. He had been scuba diving since he was ten years old. The whole family at that time became qualified scuba divers. He was very good at it and very careful. Eventually, I came to terms with his death by thinking, 'Well, he died doing what he loved.' But it was so unexpected that the whole family was in terrible shock. He left a wife and two children. He was 62 years old, but he was in good health up until the time he died. We were all in shock and disbelief. Family and friends were in a fog about losing Joseph in this manner. He did not do risky things, and he never would have continued scuba diving if he knew he was ill. No one had any knowledge otherwise. He looked and seemed very healthy."

**Penny** continued, "As I said, it was a bitterly painful experience for me and the rest of the family. Eventually, we all had to accept that Joseph died. I think my eventual growth came from realizing that Joseph had a happy life and that he died doing the activity he loved the most. Also, he wasn't in an accident or running out of oxygen while he was under the sea; his heart simply gave out. There was nothing wrong with his equipment, and he was not in dangerous circumstances. He would have died no matter what he was doing, and he loved scuba diving so much. It was his passion. His wife and kids feel the same way I do, but it was still a horrible shock, and we all miss him so much. Parents are not supposed to outlive their children and here I am in my 90s."

**Mother**: Joan
**Child**: Ryan

"My son accidentally overdosed on pain medication. He had chronic back pain for several years after a car accident. His girlfriend found him dead on the floor in the kitchen when she came home from work. It was a terrible shock for all of us. Ryan was doing so well in his new job, and they were making wedding plans. It was just a horrible shock."

"The police thought it might be suicide, but I didn't believe that because everything in his life was going very well. He had everything to live for. When he was having severe back pain, I knew he took strong pain medicine. As far as I know, his medications were prescribed by doctors; I don't think he bought drugs on the street. I miss him so much."

"At first, I felt numb and simply could not believe that he was gone. The support of family and friends has lifted me over the years. I also take solace in knowing that Ryan's death was accidental and not intentional. He was happy in his job and with his life. He had so much to look forward to. The back pain did keep him from doing some things, but he seemed to have it under control. I find comfort in thinking that Ryan died a happy man. I draw strength from knowing that he was happy."

**Grandmother**: Janet
**Grandchild**: Dana

"My granddaughter, Dana, was born on 12/25/2018. My daughter, Marian, was at 41 weeks of pregnancy when her water broke, but she did not progress in labor. She was post-term with an almost nine-pound baby, so they did a c-section delivery at 1:40 AM. The baby was beautiful and had a full head of hair. I went home to sleep because I was with my daughter at the hospital for the birth. My husband and I drove to New Jersey. My daughter was an accountant in NYC."

**Janet** stated, "I remember that Marian had professional pictures of the baby taken soon after she was born. The photographer came in for a photoshoot. I didn't say anything but remember thinking, 'Why doesn't she just get the hospital photos for now and get the professional ones later.' But I didn't say anything because this is what she wanted; it seemed important to her. I think she spent over $300 for this photo shoot."

**Janet** reported, "The baby had an increased bilirubin count when she came home from the hospital, and the pediatrician was watching it at three days of age. They came home on Friday, and the baby was doing well. On Saturday, another bilirubin test was done. Also, my daughter had gotten this device called an "Owlet Smart Sock," which was on one of the baby's feet to monitor her temperature and heart rate. It is not endorsed by the American Medical Association, but it seemed to be popular with new parents. My daughter mentioned to me that the beeper or warning device on this monitor kept going off during the night and they kept checking on the baby to make sure she was warm enough. Marian had hooked up this device to her cell phone. Her milk had come in pretty fast, so she was nursing the baby a lot and giving her skin-to-skin contact."

Janet added, "Dana had darker skin because her father, Chase, is African American. This made it harder to tell if she was jaundiced, but we relied on the bilirubin checks. Family and friends visited the new family. My daughter noticed that as the day went on the baby appeared more lethargic and started to have grunting as she was breathing. We realized that 'something was not right with the baby.' Also, we live one hour from the hospital. My house is in a very rural area. The on-call RN at the pediatrician's office told us to bring the baby to the ER at the hospital right away. We set out in my car with Chase in the front seat with me and Marian with Dana in the back seat. We were about halfway to the hospital when Marian screamed that the baby had stopped breathing. I pulled the car over to the side of the road and 'went into nurse mode.' I started doing CPR on my granddaughter. I told Chase to call 911 for an ambulance. Marian was only five days post c-section. She started screaming, 'Mom save her, Mom save her.' I didn't feel that the seat of the car was a firm enough surface for CPR after starting it, so I moved her to the back of the car with the hatchback up, which was firmer. Pretty quickly an ambulance arrived and six people were helping us. A nurse practitioner from the NICU stopped to help as well. I guess she was driving by on the road and saw us. There were EMTs from the ambulance who took over for me doing CPR and trying to stabilize the baby. Marian was screaming, and Chase was in shock. They went in the ambulance with the baby. Once they left, I remember putting my head on the steering wheel and crying. Then, I called my husband on my cell phone and told him that the baby went into cardiac arrest. A second ambulance pulled up and took me to the hospital. They told me not to drive being so upset and stressed out. At the hospital, they continued to work on saving the baby. It seemed like a long time, but I think it was only about 20 minutes. Marian told me that someone was asking for insurance information, but he turned out to be a chaplain, and he was no help. I remember my daughter saying to me later, 'Why didn't they tell me that they were sending a chaplain to talk to us?'

Janet continued, "Dana's death was considered a coroner's case because she died on the way to the hospital. We went through about three hours of questioning. No one knew that I was a nurse. It was weird because the people in the ER didn't look us in the eye if you know what I mean. Also, no one said, 'I'm sorry.' There were no kind words or anything. This added to Marian's distress. I didn't want to say anything, but we may have looked different to the personnel in the ER because Chase was African American, and Marian and Chase were not married."

Janet stated, "The coroner's assistant was the one person who reached out to us. She was amazing in the way she gathered mementos for Marian from Dana that could later be put in a shadow box, like a piece of Dana's hair. This person showed empathy and caring."

Janet continued, "Marian had a pretty normal pregnancy, but she was Group B Strep + (GBS+) and was treated with antibiotics. She also had respiratory syncytial virus (RSV) when she was pregnant, which she thought she got from her young niece and nephew, but she received treatment. The baby's autopsy report said that she died of hepatic necrosis. I guess her bilirubin levels had been high because of a necrotic liver. She had pathological hyperbilirubinemia. They told Marian that she should have genetic testing before she has another child and to make sure there was not an Rh incompatibility. Marian says that she does not want to have children after this experience."

**Janet** added, "To make a long story short, Marian has had a tough time. After losing Dana, she and Chase split up but stayed in touch. He moved to Alabama to work for his uncle. Before losing Dana, Marian planned to join him in Alabama. Chase had given Marian a dog to keep her company after losing Dana. To add to the pain, Chase was murdered in Alabama by a drive-by shooting. I think he was in the wrong place at the wrong time. It may have been that he got in with the wrong crowd of people in Alabama. Then, the dog that Chase had given Marian died. So, Marian had all these losses within a relatively short amount of time. I feel for her. Lately, she seems to be doing better but it has been a lot for one person to have. Fortunately, she has the support of her two sisters and the rest of the family and friends."

**Mother**: Barbie
**Child**: Jack

"I was on the train on my way into NYC to meet a friend for dinner. While on the train I received a call from my son, Jack, who had recently relocated to South Carolina from Florida. He was very pleased with the house he was having expanded, and it was on quite a large parcel of land near a lake. He was looking forward to having a family reunion. We had a very nice conversation on the phone. It was brief but nice. And the last thing he said to me was, 'I love you, Mom.' It was great and then the next morning about 10 AM, I received a call from a lawyer. Jack had recently been involved in a divorce action, and he had to fight for it. It was finally granted two months before. So, the first thing the lawyer said to me was, 'This is 'so and so,' Do you know that Jack was killed this morning?' I don't know how you would characterize that statement, maybe harsh, whatever? It was certainly shocking! No one had called me yet. I said, 'Are you sure?' I asked him to check with the police to make sure this information was accurate. A call had gone out to his newly divorced wife. So, that started a chain of events. Pretty soon, the lawyer called me back and confirmed the information. Jack had died walking along a road. His vehicle was being repaired at the time, and he was walking along a road and was hit by a truck. In conversations with the police, I was asking nurse-like questions in terms of identification. One of the officers said to me that he was not recognizable facially, but they were able to confirm his identity through a tattoo along with some of the papers he had with him. It happened in the early morning, so it was somewhat dark. It was a large truck, and I think the truck driver stopped. We are talking like an 18-wheeler. The information being released set off a bunch of actions. I had to notify my daughter and my younger son. Jack also had three daughters. They were adult daughters. I called his first wife who was the mother of the girls. The divorce that had just gone through was not with his first wife. The last one was a short marriage, maybe a year and a half. I didn't want to call the daughters; I wanted to check with their mother to see if she wanted to tell them. They had a good relationship (first wife), and I was the one who called her to tell her. Fortunately, this happened on March 17, St. Patrick's Day 2017, and it was the first day of my spring break. God is good, I was free in terms of time to do all these things. Then, I did speak with his first wife, and she agreed it would be appropriate if I notified their daughters. They all lived in different places and different states, so I went about getting in touch with the girls. Ironically, I was getting voice recordings, and I tried to leave a message which was not the true reason why I was calling. I emphasized that I wanted them to get in touch with me right away. That took a couple of hours until I got the three of them. Then, I had to proceed to make arrangements, and they were long-distance arrangements. My daughter, Sharon, was the executor of Jack's will, and in conversation with her, we made funeral arrangements."

**Barbie** added, "Jack, like his father, had a drinking problem but he was trying to address it, and even in our last conversation we talked about him going someplace to get a hold of himself. He was good 23 hours of the day. I have done considerable research on alcoholism and my master's thesis was on alcoholism. I have been to many events around the country focusing on the abuse of alcohol. This experience confirmed my strength, organization, take-charge attitude, and my consideration for others. I couldn't do anything to bring my son back, but I wanted to give him a proper funeral and a ceremony or celebration of his life. I'm glad that Jack and I had that last conversation."

**Mother**: Carla
**Child**: Cassandra

"Part of myself died when Cassandra was killed in the plane crash. I knew in that instant that my life would never be the same. How do you ever get over losing a child? It is against the natural order of things. She was fine and happy one day and dead the next. It was a terrible accident that took two young lives, leaving two families heartbroken. It has affected me every day, and it has been several years."

**Carla** continued, "The early days were the worst because we were in shock. I still think about Cassandra and her love of flying. I try to tell myself that she died doing what she truly loved." Carla added, "I also feel extremely protective of my younger daughter Bernadette. She had such a tough time losing her sister, who was her best friend. Her grades suffered, she had anxiety and depression, and she felt lost without Cassandra. Bernadette is very close to me and her father. She relies on us a lot. We thank God for her. But why did God have to take Cassandra away from us at such a young age? We will always be heartbroken."

*Anticipated Loss*

**Mother**: Diane
**Child**: Darren

"Darren was diagnosed with a brain tumor at three years of age. For the next ten years, he went through numerous treatments for it in NYC. He had chemotherapy, radiation, and surgery. He was never 'cured,' but it was 'managed.' We had good years and bad years. He finally passed away at 13. He was a fighter, and it was a roller-coaster ride for our family. Darren was the best son ever and hardly ever complained. He made us stronger as a family. Darren enriched our family life. We appreciated life so much because he did. We have been able to keep that feeling going because he inspired us immensely. We took a lot of family vacations, and they were awesome. Darren brought us so much joy in those 13 years. He taught us so much too, about bravery, courage, spirituality, and love. We continue to feel 'blessed' as a family and Darren left such an imprint on our lives. His strength gave us strength. He brought out the best in people and brought everyone closer. Our immediate family and our extended family of aunts and uncles, cousins, family friends, his classmates, and everyone he came in contact with, including the nurses and doctors at the hospital, feel like they are better people for having Darren in their lives."

**Diane** continued, "I think both family and friends are closer because of Darren. He had that effect on people. Plus, we learned to ask for help and accept help in difficult times. He was a brave boy and brought out bravery and courage in others. With two other kids, we knew we had to keep going. Darren's death was hard on everyone, but we all feel like better people because of him. He brought out the best in everyone."

**Mother**: Gloria
**Child**: Alice

"My pregnancy was uneventful, and then at 27 weeks I went into premature labor, and I delivered a set of female twins by cesarean section. One twin weighed 1 pound 13 ounces, and the other twin weighed 1 pound 7 ounces. They were in the Neonatal Intensive Care Unit (NICU) for about five and a half months. It was a rollercoaster for several months, and Alice never made it out of the NICU. Alice had severe respiratory depression and remained on a ventilator the entire time she was in the NICU. Her lungs were very immature, and no matter what the neonatology team did it didn't seem to help that much. There were good days and bad days. Lara had neurological problems, but I was able to finally take her home at about five and a half months. She had a tracheostomy for about five years to help her breathe. Fortunately, I had the babies at a large children's hospital in the city, and I was working at the time myself for the College of Medicine in the Division of Neonatology. So, when I went back to work at about three weeks which seems very early, it allowed me to go up and see the babies several times during my workday. The doctors didn't know specifically why I went into premature labor although, with my first pregnancy with my daughter, I was on bed rest because my cervix started to thin out and I had to stop working at 39 weeks. The other reason that might have had something to do with the premature labor, but they weren't sure was that my mother died four days before I went into premature labor with the twins. There may have been a connection with my emotional distress about losing my mother. Also, carrying a twin pregnancy puts you more at risk for premature labor anyway. I was not able to go to my mother's funeral on the east coast, but my husband went. My friend, Delores, came and stayed with me so that I could remain on bed rest at home with the twins. Alice passed away in the NICU a few days after we brought Lara home. Somehow, we managed, but I have to say that it was very difficult."

**Mother**: Colleen
**Child**: Max

"Max was 42 years old at the time of his death. He had heart problems since childhood, and they became worse as he got older. He went into the hospital on July 9 and never got out. I urged him to go to the hospital, and so did his brothers because his feet were extremely swollen. He looked like Bigfoot. He was also sweating a lot and felt weak. He was the type of guy who would never tell you if he wasn't feeling well; he would just say that he was 'okay.' He first went to the local community hospital, and then they transferred him to a big medical center in Boston by helicopter. After being at that medical center, they transferred him to another one across town. Days later they transferred him back to the original medical center where his cardiologist practiced. She insisted that he be at her facility. He had gone to this same specialist for most of his life. She studied the genetic condition that Max had. I don't know why there was all this transferring between hospitals except that they were trying to get him the best care with the best people. They said he was 'critical but stable,' whatever that means. Eventually, Max had a cardiac arrest. Later, he had a blood clot in his brain. He was on life support, and we had to decide to take him off because there was no hope of recovery. It was so hard (crying). He was the best kid. He'd give you the shirt off his back. He was that kind of person."

**Colleen** added, "They say that parents are supposed to go first and children later. It's so hard to lose a child, to bury a child. Even when your child is an adult, it is still so hard because they are still your child no matter how old they are. It was tough because Max was such a beautiful person. I know that I'm a strong person, but it still hurts. I think my coping has improved a bit over time, but it is still very painful. They tried to give me medication for anxiety and depression, but I refused. I didn't think I needed it. I'd rather just cope in my way. I think I may experience more growth in the future. I guess I've had some growth if I'm able to go on and not need medication. But it still hurts so much to think about Max and what he went through. He lived with me, so it's apparent to me every day that he is not there. We were close and he was always helpful."

**Grandmother**: Jean
**Grandchild**: Amy

"In 2011, I was going to be a grandmother for the first time. It was my son and daughter-in-law who live about three miles away from me. At 23 weeks of pregnancy, my daughter-in-law had an ultrasound and was told that the baby had a cardiac abnormality referred to as a hypoplastic left heart. It was devastating to me. 'It broke my heart, and I could feel my heart shatter in my chest.' Being in health care, I knew that this was a serious abnormality and that it would affect the child's life greatly. Because it was still fairly early in the pregnancy, the doctor advised my daughter-in-law and son to terminate the pregnancy. They felt differently and had the mindset that God blessed them with this baby and that they would do everything possible to give the baby the best chance at life. They did their homework and investigated research through the American Heart Association. I decided to play the devil's advocate and give them an idea of what the struggles and challenges would be in the future. As a healthcare provider, I wondered if the termination was the right thing to do, and I felt awful about it, but I had a pretty good idea of what these parents would face in the future with a sick child. I also knew that there was a chance that the baby would not survive in the long run. It was an ethical dilemma, a sad and worrisome situation, and the news broke all our hearts."

"They decided to go on with the pregnancy, and at 31 weeks my daughter-in-law had a spontaneous rupture of membranes and was hospitalized for four to five weeks to let the baby continue to grow and the lungs mature. At about 33 weeks, she went into labor and delivered a baby girl with a left hypoplastic heart. They named her Amy. She was born at a large medical center in NYC that had a Neonatal Intensive Care Unit (NICU). Even though she would need open-heart surgery, it was the policy to wait until the baby is five pounds at this medical center. The plan was to have three cardiac procedures over three years, and basically, the child lives with a two-chamber heart. Besides the hypoplastic left heart, the baby had a syndrome referred to as VACTERL. VACTERL is a disorder that can affect many body parts. VACTERL stands for vertebral defects, anal atresia, cardiac defects, trachea-esophageal fistula, renal abnormalities, and limb abnormalities. Most VACTERL babies have at least three of these defects. Supposedly, its cause is an interaction of multiple genetic and environmental factors. The developmental abnormalities develop before birth."

"The NICU team focused on the quality of life with intubation, followed by the first surgery which was to focus on the trachea-esophageal atresia. Then, there was a second surgery which was a colostomy because there was also duodenal atresia. The baby was getting TPN (total parenteral nutrition) through a special type of intravenous line for nutrition. I saw myself as an advocate for my granddaughter and her parents. Although sometimes I felt like everyone around me wanted me to keep my mouth shut. The third surgery was the open-heart surgery, and we were told that she did very well."

**Jean** continued, "I remember coming home from the hospital to eat and sleep. Later, I received a telephone call from my son who was screaming, 'She's dead, she's dead!' When he calmed down, he said that Amy was doing all right, and the nurses told them to go and take a shower in their room and get some rest. They came back from showering and were told that Amy died. There was no other explanation except that she passed away after surgery, which they knew could happen. It was just awful. I went back to the hospital, and this was the first chance I got to hold my granddaughter. I wish more could have been done for her. I have a 'Memory Box' that still has her receiving blanket in it with her blood on it. I will keep it forever. My son and daughter-in-law were in such pain, and so was I. Amy was my first grandchild. I still have such a mix of emotions, but I can talk about it. I don't mind talking to people about it. I think it helps me."

**Jean** added, "Now, my son and daughter-in-law have two wonderful sons. It's been eight years, and I still think about Amy. Lee is now six years old and loves to ice skate and is on a hockey team. Harry is 18 months and a very busy little guy. Between the two boys were two failed IVF attempts, and Harry was born prematurely at 34 weeks and was in the same NICU in NYC where Amy died."

**Mother**: Chantelle
**Child**: Mark

**Chantelle** reported, "My oldest son died of kidney failure when he was 45 years old. They offered to put him on the kidney transplant list, but he refused because he would not give up smoking cigarettes. They will not give someone a kidney transplant if they smoke cigarettes or have a drinking problem or are taking drugs. His stubbornness and lack of motivation kept him from living or having a chance to continue living. Mark was a rebel even as a child. He always did what he wanted to do and would not listen to the advice of others (teachers, policemen, coaches, doctors, or his parents). He would always say, 'No one is going to tell me what to do.' For most of his adult life when he was not in jail,

Mark would live on the streets or sometimes in his car, if he had one at the time. He lived like this for at least ten years and didn't keep in touch with me very often. I heard from him more often toward the end of his life. Then, one night I got a call from his girlfriend in the middle of the night saying that he was in the hospital. She said that he was taken to the hospital by ambulance because he was acting incoherently. She said that he appeared to be very sick. He had been on dialysis for some time because of kidney problems, and that week he had missed one or two appointments because 'He didn't feel like going.' I think he had picked up hepatitis while he was in jail, too. His health had not been good for about ten years. He ended up with methicillin-resistant *Staphylococcus aureus* (MRSA) in the hospital and was very sick. He never regained consciousness."

**Chantelle** shared, "As a mother, it was very frustrating because Mark did not take care of himself. I tried everything including 'tough love' and a bunch of other things, but nothing seemed to work. He left our home when he was in his early 20s after I told him that he had to 'get out.' I had to do this because I was widowed and had three other kids. I was afraid that he would influence them and get them into trouble. I didn't know what else to do at the time. My husband and I had taken Mark to see doctors and psychologists about his bad behavior when he was younger. He had problems in school. The medications, counseling, and 'tough love' did not work. He didn't follow through with anything and simply wanted to do what he wanted to do. This was so frustrating for everyone involved."

"I did see Mark occasionally in the last few years when he was out of jail. I did not like his girlfriend because I didn't feel that she was a good influence on him. Within a few weeks of his death, she had a new boyfriend. That was 'goodbye' to her which was fine with me."

**Mother**: Ellen
**Child**: Jane

"In 2005, when I was 20 weeks pregnant, I found out that my daughter had a right heart abnormality, and then she was diagnosed later with DiGeorge syndrome. She was delivered at 37 1/2 weeks by c-section at a large medical center in NYC. She was supposed to have surgery when she was two weeks old. She did great initially, but we knew she had serious surgical complications. She had an 8 mm hole in her heart. She scored high mentally, and her other tests were good. They rushed her into surgery at five days of age. The aorta had stunted growth, and the pulmonary artery was very enlarged. They tried four times to patch her heart, but she suffered brain, kidney, and liver failure. So, they just closed her up. She had surgery on 9/5 and she died at 4 AM on 9/7."

"I remember seeing a geneticist at 22 weeks. It was not a good experience. This doctor advised me to abort my daughter. He was not professional or humanistic or sensitive in any way. He focused on everything negative. I told him that as long as my daughter was fighting for her life, I would fight for her life, too. He said that I had only one week to decide whether to terminate or they'd have to send me to another state. He showed me a picture of what she would look like, and that this syndrome has up to 176 symptoms. I could not believe it. I was in shock, mostly about his behavior. He assumed that if she wasn't 100% perfect, I wouldn't want her."

"Originally, my doctor's office said that my amniocentesis was fine except for the noted problem with her heart. Then, the doctor told me that she had DiGeorge syndrome, which ranged in symptoms from ADD (attention deficit disorder) to serious heart problems. After checking with the amnio report and the other associated tests, my doctor called me to tell me that she had very serious heart problems and that she may not live. I remember him saying that 'pediatric cardiologists think that they can fix everything, they think that everything they touch turns to gold and that simply is not true.' He kept repeating, 'This is very serious and I'm telling you that your daughter could die.' He said, 'I am trying to prepare you for the decisions you will be facing. There is a good chance that she won't make it. You have a very sick child.' I remember him saying, 'I'm praying for you, I'm fighting with you, but I want you to be prepared.'"

"After this phone call, my doctor called me every day for the next 10 1/2 weeks to check in on me. He was a great guy. After Jane died, I returned to see my doctor at six weeks and eight weeks postpartum. He wanted to keep tabs on how I was doing. At the end of my six-week postpartum visit, he showed me a prayer card from her funeral. He said he carries it with him all the time. He said that it makes him a better doctor, a better man, and a better person. He advised me to wait one year before getting pregnant again so that I would be in a better place. He wanted me to mourn, heal, and give myself time before facing another pregnancy. I waited one year to the day. He delivered my fourth child. He is an amazing man. He's still involved at the hospital. He wants to keep his hand in."

**Ellen** continued, "Each one of my pregnancies got worse and worse, and worse. I've had hemorrhages and been hooked up to IVs. When my daughter died, if my water broke, I would have been in serious trouble. I had polyhydramnios with about 55 cm of amniotic fluid at 37 weeks. It was the right decision to do a c-section birth at 37 1/2 weeks at a large medical center in NYC rather than at a community hospital. I was scared but I didn't want to leave my kids motherless."

## Theme: When I Lost My Child, I Lost Part of Myself

The women described their emotions in coming to terms with their devastating loss. Initially, everyone wondered how they could go on with their lives. Even when death was probable given the prognosis, a ray of hope remained. No one could easily shut the door on their loved one. The happy memories of the child remained, and they held them tightly in their heart and mind. However, the women had a sense of loss, an emptiness, and a void in their lives. The following quotations give testimony to this theme.

**Carla**: "When Cassandra was killed in the plane crash, I knew that my life would never be the same. It was as if part of me died when she died. I didn't know how I could go on without her. She was my firstborn. She was a delight, a simply wonderful daughter. She had such a bright future ahead of her. As a family, we had so much to look forward to. I wondered how this could happen to us. What would become of us without Cassandra? I knew the void would be so painful. I questioned how God could allow this to happen to our family. With her death, I felt like a piece of my heart was cut out of my body. At times, I felt numb in the months to follow. My husband threw all his being into his work. I think he kept so busy that he would not think about the loss. Work was his escape. My sadness overwhelmed me, and I think I functioned much like a robot or a zombie. The first three years were the worst."

**Susan**: "My husband and I were in such a state of shock to think that our beautiful daughter committed suicide over a break-up with her boyfriend. We wished she had told us of her hurt and disappointment. We would have listened and offered support and love.

We felt sad, lost, guilty, and a host of other emotions. Our hearts were broken, but we still had so many unanswered questions. We surmised that Brianne took the bottle of pills in a fit of rage, anger, hurt, and disappointment. We wondered if we'd ever have answers to our questions. It was like a horrible dream."

**Colleen**: "I've been through death before, but when it's your kid, it is the hardest. He was such a good kid, too. Sometimes I feel like I'll never get over losing Max, but they say that time helps. I think I have a few more years to go."

**Gloria**: "I guess I always knew that it could be 'touch and go' with premature twins. Although I knew that they could both have deficits, I was hopeful when we finally got to take Lara home after such a long time in the NICU. I prayed that Alice would follow her sister into our home eventually, but her lungs were never strong enough to survive and make it out of the NICU. It was heartbreaking that she didn't survive after fighting for her life for so many months. As devastated as we were, we had to go on for the sake of Lara and our older daughter."

**Joan**: "I think it was the element of shock and disbelief that knocked me for a loop. Ryan was at a high point in his life; he was successful in his career and planning a wedding. This was not supposed to happen. It was a nightmare for me because I thought he was clean, off drugs for pain. This had to be a horrible accident because he did not intend to kill himself. I have so many unanswered questions and they'll never be answered."

**Janet**: "Dana was my first grandchild and supposedly there was nothing wrong with her when she came home from the hospital. We did all the right things until my daughter noticed she was deteriorating over a day or two. As a nurse, my daughter looked to me to save her as we were driving to the hospital. I stopped the car and initiated CPR until the ambulance crew came and took over. When they told us at the hospital that Dana 'didn't make it,' I was heartbroken both for myself and my daughter. The hurt and sense of loss were compounded by all the questioning that we went through. I guess they had to ask questions because Dana died before reaching the hospital. As a healthcare professional, I know that these occurrences must be investigated. However, the people in the ER could have been kinder to the three of us. Unfortunately, there seemed to be a lack of sensitivity and empathy except for one person who talked to us. This is what I remember."

**Barbie**: "Jack had a few tough years before he was hit by the truck. However, he seemed to be doing better. My shock and disbelief added to my pain. It was so sudden, and I had just had a nice conversation with him. The police questioned whether he purposely walked out in front of the truck, but I don't believe this. It was dark outside and on a very poorly lit country road. I just think it was a terrible accident. You know, being in the wrong place at the wrong time. That's how accidents happen sometimes. My heart sank in my chest, and then I had to contact the family and plan the funeral."

**Ellen**: "Losing Jane was the hardest thing my husband and I had ever experienced. Because of the situation and the advice of the maternal–fetal medicine experts, her birth was a planned c-section delivery at a renowned NYC medical center with a pediatric team ready to evaluate her as soon as she entered the world. We wanted to give her the best shot at life, and I think in the long run that is exactly what we did. However, God wanted Jane with Him. Our strong faith understood this, but we still experienced an immense and devastating loss. I had fought so hard for this baby. Our hearts were broken even though we knew prenatally that Jane had worrisome health problems. You hate to give up hope because that hope had kept you going for so long."

**Diane**: "We had so many ups and downs with Darren's cancer, but we never gave up hope. He was an inspiration to all of us. He was our firstborn and the light of our lives. Still to this day, I don't know how we were able to go on living without him. But when you have other children that need you, you must go on for them. My husband and I know that Darren had the best care, and we were his strongest advocates and his cheerleaders. Everyone loved him; he was a great kid."

### Theme: Picking Up the Pieces of My Life

Participants shared their struggles and triumphs. There were some examples of posttraumatic growth in their lives, such as joining organizations such as Compassionate Friends, the March of Dimes, and Sisters of Heart. Some sought individual therapy, and others did group therapy. Some women participated in bereavement groups at churches, hospitals, and community organizations. Many benefited from grief counseling and other types of support. Many reflected sentiments of knowing that they were not alone and that others had similar losses. Many women kept busy caring for other children or returned to work, which served as a bit of a distraction or necessity. While attending to the details of their lives, many women expressed a gradual appreciation of life.

**Janet**: "I believe that Dana's short life had a purpose. My therapist told me, 'You are dealing with it, and you are growing from the experience.' I think I have posttraumatic growth. One sign of it was that I was able to teach my nursing students about perinatal loss. In the beginning, I simply could not do it. I had another faculty member cover that content. But when we were dealing with Covid-19, I was able to finally do it. That was a milestone for me. Overall, work was a blessing. It is healthy to surround yourself with supportive, positive people. My nursing colleagues tend to be nurturing people; we pick each other up when needed. I know that I have been there for others when they encountered difficult circumstances and when I needed them, they were there for me."

**Janet** added, "To make a long story short, Marian has had a tough time. After losing Dana, she and Chase split up but stayed in touch. He moved to Alabama to work for his uncle. Before losing Dana, Marian planned to join him in Alabama. Chase had given Marian a dog to keep her company after losing Dana. To add to the pain, Chase was murdered in Alabama by a drive-by shooting. I think he was in the wrong place at the wrong time. It may have been that he got in with the wrong crowd of people in Alabama. Then, the dog that Chase had given Marian died. So, Marian had all these losses within a relatively short amount of time. I feel for her. Lately, she seems to be doing better, but it has been a lot for one person to have. Fortunately, she has the support of her two sisters and the rest of her family and friends.

**Amanda**: "Joining Compassionate Friends and eventually becoming a co-leader with another woman who had lost a daughter helped me pick up the pieces of my life. For me, I got a lot from being with others who had lost a child. There was camaraderie, friendship, and a sense of belonging without having to reiterate every detail of your life. There was openness, acceptance, and honesty at the meetings. You never felt compelled to talk if you did not want to share. There was not a sense of pressure to tell your story. Every person must find their way of dealing with loss just as they have to find their way of living their life."

**Jean**: "After losing Amy, I had PTSD. I went into therapy, which helped a lot. I used my pain in positive ways. I became very active in the March of Dimes and have kept this up for the last eight years. I also joined an organization called 'Sisters by Heart,' and I have knitted over 4,000 baby hats for these little ones. I even put a snap in the hat in case the baby has an IV line in its scalp. I found a way to make my pain work for me. I would share this with other bereaved parents and grandparents. What I took away from this sad, devastating experience were many positives. For example, I am now more accepting of people; I want to help people in any way that I can. I have been able to 'soul search' and reflect. 'I try to be the best that I can be because of Amy.' I stopped wearing a watch after Amy died because time didn't matter as much as it did before. I also joined a Grandparent's Bereavement Group. We meet online because it would be over a 90-minute drive for me to get to a meeting. I tell my two grandsons that they are 'Rainbow Babies' because their sister was born before they were and that she is in heaven."

**Diane**: "With two other children who were younger than Darren, I had to get my act together quickly because life kept going with kids in school. I think the kids' activities, their homework, and my husband's job dominated our family life. Of course, there was a big hole in our hearts after Darren died. We had faith in God, a supportive extended family, and monetary resources. Our financial stability allowed us to take vacations to Disney World, go to a beach resort, or go on a cruise. Many families don't have the means to do these things. These distractions served a purpose for us, in that they helped the kids have a change of scenery, have new adventures, and do fun things. After losing Darren, we all needed an occasional vacation. My husband and I benefitted as much as the kids did."

**Susan**: "After Brianne's suicide, my husband and I felt that we had to be strong for our other children. We had to explain things and answer a lot of questions because she was our oldest and a freshman in college. The kids had trouble relating to the fact that their sister was so sad that she decided to take her own life. We were honest with the kids and tried not to sugarcoat things. The break-up with Jason shattered Brianne's world to the extent that she took a bottle of pills. It was an impulsive, angry act done in haste. He was her first serious boyfriend and I guess she could not imagine her life without having him in it. She was an emotional girl, a perfectionist, and a straight-A student. However, she was also inexperienced, immature, and a very concrete thinker."

**Susan** added, "We had to keep going as a family because there were obligations, such as school, sports, and church. My husband dove right back into his work while I tried to do the usual things at home. Both of us read everything we could get our hands on about suicide and depression. We wanted to be alert and informed for the sake of our kids in case they had similar issues in the future."

**Carla**: "We were in a state of shock, disbelief, and numbness for what seemed like a long time. We were also guilt-ridden for letting Cassandra get her pilot's license. But she was a safe, organized, and talented pilot. How could we keep her from doing something she loved so much? I was a zombie and on a perpetual treadmill for a long time after the accident. I had no job to go back to and was not in the frame of mind to look for one. I knew that with another child to raise, I could not stay in bed all day or drink wine all day or engage in my shopaholic behavior nonstop. I had to be there for our middle schooler, attend sporting events, teach religious education at church, cook evening meals, and function as a responsible adult. Yet, part of me didn't want to do any of these things. I just wanted to stay in bed and pull the covers over my head and feel sorry for myself. For the first year, I cried every day. I missed Cassandra so much. The whole experience was a nightmare, but I had to put on 'my game face' for the sake of my family and friends. Plus, when you have the responsibility for another child, you must go on living. Parental obligations and responsibilities run deep, and with God's help, I was able to continue to be there for Bernadette. She needed me because she had lost her best friend, her older sister, Cassandra. They were close, thick as thieves, partners in crime. They were 'Thelma and Louise' personified. So, I sought to help Bernadette in any way possible. Her happiness became my life's mission."

**Gloria**: "When Alice died in the NICU, we already had brought Lara home. So, we had to just keep going. We had no choice. Of course, we were sad and disappointed. Our dream of having twin girls with a doting big sister vanished in a heartbeat. Also, Lara had numerous health problems, and her care was involved and time-consuming. We knew that we were fortunate to have one surviving twin, but losing Alice after almost six months in the NICU was heartbreaking. You keep hoping and praying that these little ones will survive, but intellectually you know that it might not be the case. We got help to care for Lara, so I eventually returned to work, which was therapeutic for me. I liked my work, and because I worked at a hospital, it put me in touch with the best specialists for Lara. My co-workers were phenomenal, which made such a positive difference in my life because my small family lived on the east coast and my mother had died when I was pregnant with the twins."

**Gloria** added, "After losing Alice the only thing that changed was not going to the NICU to see her. We had Lara home with us, and she needed a lot of care. I think my husband and I had been on automatic pilot for so long with two premature babies in the NICU that we just went through the motions of life. We also had our older daughter at home and we both had to work. Also, Lara had so many doctor's appointments and therapy appointments because of her cerebral palsy and tracheostomy. I just kept juggling responsibilities, and everyone was kind, patient, and caring. Although we felt the loss we had to move on. Those months with both babies in the NICU were a roller coaster ride with some hopeful days and other worrisome days. There was so much uncertainty and so many prayers. We knew from the start that Alice and Lara might not survive; that we might not bring them home."

**Gloria** continued, "When Lara survived, my life took on a major advocacy role for her. They said that she'd never walk, but with lots of physical therapy, she can walk. Sure, she tires easily and uses a wheelchair, when necessary, but she can walk. She doesn't have a tracheostomy anymore. I stay on top of things for her. In today's healthcare system, everyone needs an advocate. Lara has come a long way."

**Colleen**: "My third son, Max, died of an inherited heart defect at age 42. He was such a beautiful person. At first, I thought I would never be able to move past his death, but when others depend on you it's hard not to be there for them. That's what I did for my three other kids. I kept working part-time, too, because we needed the money."

**Colleen** added, "Max's death was the hardest in my life, and I've had several of them. It was so strange when Max was gone. He was missed every day by all of us. We were constantly reminded of him everywhere we looked. Although he lived with a serious cardiac defect, he had many good days until the last few months. I don't think I'll ever be 100% again without Max in my life. He was that special."

**Penny**: "When Joe died while scuba diving, I couldn't just think about my loss, I had to think about the loss of my son as a husband and father, too. His wife and children were devastated. We were all in shock. We were close, but we grew even closer. We gained strength from each other."

**Penny** added, "Being a widow, I had a better idea of what my daughter-in-law was going through. My family, friends, and people from church were there for all of us. These resources helped me get my life back on track. I've always been a strong and independent woman, but as I get older, I live more in the moment."

**Penny** continued, "As I said, it was a bitterly painful experience for me and the rest of the family. Eventually, we all had to accept that Joseph died. I think my eventual growth came from realizing that Joseph had a happy life and that he died doing the activity he loved the most. Also, he wasn't in an accident or running out of oxygen while he was under the sea; his heart simply gave out. There was nothing wrong with his equipment, and he was not in dangerous circumstances. He would have died no matter what he was doing, and he loved scuba diving so much. It was his passion. His wife and kids feel the same way I do, but it was still a horrible shock, and we all miss him so much. Parents are not supposed to outlive their children, and here I am in my 90s."

**Joan**: "I still believe that Ryan's death was an accidental overdose. I admit that I was disappointed that he still occasionally was involved with recreational drugs. I don't think he was trying to kill himself. I miss him, his fiancée misses him, his friends miss him, and his siblings miss him."

**Chantelle**: "I was angry and disappointed that Mark chose to continue smoking cigarettes, which kept him from being placed on the list for a kidney transplant. We were not surprised when he died of end-stage renal disease. We went on with our lives but felt very frustrated and disappointed with Mark's choice." Chantelle continued, "I could not let the negative emotions take over my life because I had other kids. My life was always a struggle financially, but I always put one foot in front of the other and moved on."

**Ellen**: "Eventually, I think I had some posttraumatic growth. I had my phases of mourning and healing. I knew I had to be strong for my other kids. All my kids have had health problems. I think I have been stronger because of what I went through with Jane. My older daughter keeps me grounded these days. I have been through significant problems with both sons having surgery. I seem to have this calm inner strength that I didn't have before I lost Jane. With all my kids having health problems, I've needed to have a calm mind."

### Theme: Support, Kindness, and Compassion Helped

None of the women participating in the study expressed a lack of support, kindness, or compassion. They mentioned family, friends, co-workers, healthcare professionals, and clergy. Many declared that they had the desire to help others after going through their experience of loss. For some, it became their new mission in life as a tribute to their loved ones. They wanted to honor the person they lost by 'paying it forward,' so to speak. They viewed this as a way to thank others for their kindness, help, support, and compassion.

**Gloria** continued, "I realized that I was a lot stronger than I thought I was. After this experience, I feel that I give attention to people whom I might not have given attention to before. I want to help people, and I want to be there for people. I think a lot of this may have come from Lara's outcome with her neurological deficits. I met a lot of people in that process because she needed a lot of help and had so many therapy appointments and doctors' appointments and surgeries. I saw a lot of other people who needed help when I was going through this with Lara over the years."

**Gloria** shared, "My sense of compassion grew, and I have more empathy for people. After what I had been through all these things stayed with me and I think that's why I'm a positive person today. I have a lot of understanding of people in difficult circumstances. I try to look on the bright side and my glass is always half full, not half empty."

**Gloria** remarked, "I've become much more assertive in dealing with all the doctors and professionals over the years. I'm a strong advocate for Lara. I've had to do my homework and ask the right questions. At times, I've had to push a bit to get what Lara needed. For example, some doctors said that she would never walk, and I thought that with the proper therapy, she would. Her therapists agreed with me. Well, Lara can walk. She may walk slower than you or me, but she can walk. She only uses a wheelchair when she's tired or when we are doing a lot of walking at the mall. I am her strongest advocate, and I guess you could say I evolved! Sometimes you surprise yourself, but you have to be a strong advocate for your child."

**Gloria** commented, "I try never to be negative. I had to push for Lara especially when I was told she probably would never walk. She walks and when she goes on a trip, we bring a wheelchair if she needs it. Today, she is on a field trip to a museum, and they bring a travel chair because it will probably involve quite a bit of walking. When she gets home, she's going for a facial. She loves that. She gets a massage every two weeks. Yes, she has quite the life! (laughing)"

**Gloria** remarked, "At the time all this was happening, our older daughter Jenna was six years old. All of this was a lot to handle for me and my husband, but fortunately, we had very good friends and colleagues as a support system. We had no family in the area: everyone was on the east coast. Because I worked at the Medical Center I had so many friends and colleagues at work who were helpful. Everyone was wonderful."

**Gloria** continued, "I appreciated all the help people gave us. I have always tried to look on the bright side of life; the glass is always half full for me. My older daughter, Jenna, and I talk about that a lot. I guess we both feel more compassionate, more caring, and more appreciative."

**Gloria** added, "My family was as supportive as they could be. My father came out to visit us and tried to help as much as he could. I have to say that we lost a few friends who simply could not deal with the fact that we had a disabled child, but you know they weren't real friends to begin with, I guess. The friends that stuck by us were great. My close friend, Anna, came out for about ten days when we brought Lara home from the hospital. I think she even visited when the twins were in the NICU. I can't exactly remember; it was a long time ago. When my mother passed away and I was on bed rest at home, my friend, Delores, came from Virginia to stay with me so that my husband could go to my mother's funeral. Later, Delores moved back from Virginia to Indiana. Delores ended up being a caregiver for Lara for about a year. She had to learn how to do trach care and everything else. At first, I think she was afraid of doing something wrong, but she watched me do it a few times and decided that she could do it. She ended up being fine with it. Delores had been a babysitter for Jenna when she was little. My first caregiver for Lara was a grandmother of a child who had a trach, so she was used to doing that type of care. This was when I first went back to work after Lara was home with us. I think I took a leave for six months at first and then I started getting people to come in."

**Colleen**: "What helped me the most was the support and kindness of my older son, Bob, his wife, and my younger son, Richard. They stayed close to me and helped with household chores, grocery shopping, and meal preparation. I did not feel alone. I feel compassion for anyone going through an ordeal like this. Your child is your child even if they are an adult. It is against the natural order of things for parents to bury their children."

**Colleen** shared, "I feel compassion for anyone going through an ordeal like this. But I also feel low on energy to deal with other people's problems, and we all have them. I try to just get by and take care of my family. I feel sad at times, but I don't want to take medication for it. I don't think I need medication; I'm coping okay. I don't think I'll ever get over Max's death. It hurts; it hurts. Life is not the same without him. Losing a child is the hardest thing a mother can face. But when you have other family members, somehow you go on. I guess I'm strong because somehow, I was able to go on living. I even quit smoking recently after many years. I think the loss of a child is the deepest hurt a parent can have. I often think of those parents whose kids were killed at that elementary school in Sandy Hook, Connecticut, and how those parents will never be the same again. And those kids were little children. Part of you dies when you lose a child no matter what their age is. Things aren't supposed to happen this way. Children are supposed to outlive their parents."

**Colleen** concluded, "I don't know if I have a philosophy of life. But what I do know is that the pain stays with you because you miss that person, and nothing can replace them. I think you have to make the best of each day and do what you are supposed to do to get by. You don't forget the person you've lost, but you have to keep going. I've had other losses in my life, but Max was the greatest. I didn't expect him to die at 42, but I knew he had heart problems all his life."

**Janet**: "I was overwhelmed with the kindness and caring of my colleagues and friends. When they learned the horrific details of what happened with my granddaughter, they eased some of my burden at work. They respected my privacy."

**Janet** commented, "My relationships with my husband and family have grown, but they were strong to begin with. I have a friend, Bernice, who is an ER nurse, who has been there for me. She is a strong, experienced nurse and a great friend. Also, my three daughters are close, and Marian is my youngest. It was a bit rocky when she was a teenager. When she was pregnant, she was amazing and happy. After the loss of Dana, she pulled back quite a bit. Now, I have a quiet presence in her life. She lets me be there."

**Chantelle**: "I was frustrated, angry, and lost when Max died of kidney failure, or as they called it 'end-stage renal disease.' He could have done things to help himself but chose not to. As a mother, I felt like I hit a brick wall. My two sons came to the rescue with their love and kindness. They gave me a lot of practical help, too. They cooked, cleaned, and did laundry."

**Susan**: "I come from a large family, and I must say that my sisters and brothers were there for us in our time of need. We felt protected, loved, listened to, and cared about. We didn't have to ask for anything, my siblings seemed to magically anticipate our needs. Cousins helped our children by being attentive, socializing, and comforting them. It is horrible to lose a child, especially to suicide. But I imagine that it can be worse if you have no one around who cares about you. Thank God, everyone banded together to be there for our family."

**Susan** shared, "I feel compassion and empathy for any parent who loses a child for any reason, but it is especially hard when it is sudden death and even more painful when it is a suicide. Parents tend to blame themselves because they are entrusted with the care of their children by God. So, when something happens there's the 'woulda, coulda, shoulda.'

Parental guilt can be plentiful, intense, and so stressful. We are always on the lookout for depression and anxiety in our other kids. I see myself as a survivor."

**Susan** added, "I believe that I became even closer to my siblings after Brianne took her own life. I think this terrible event served as a 'wake-up call' for all of us as parents. We realized that our older kids have their own lives in high school and college, and we can't be 'watchdogs' every minute. We wish we could put our kids in a protective bubble, but we know that is impossible."

**Jean**: "The most support I received was from family and friends. I must say that the organization Sisters by Heart touched my heart and soul. For a while after Amy passed away, I would say that it was challenging with heartbreak and stress. I almost thought I was resented because I was in healthcare. I knew too much, and I gave my opinion about things. I have three sons, but only one lives near me. I think my daughter-in-law, Amy's mother, sometimes resented that my son and I were close. We had a 'Come to Jesus' meeting, and now things are better. We got stuff out in the open and moved on."

**Jean** continued, "Some friends were sympathetic and understanding at first but expected me to 'get over this.' I had to explain to a few friends that this is not something that you simply 'get over.' This was my first grandchild, and I was there for all of it. As I said before, 'I was devastated and could feel my heart shatter in my chest.' Unless someone had walked in my shoes, they don't get it."

**Amanda**: "The caring, support, kindness, and compassion from friends, family, and co-workers were tremendous. We were so broken. Yet, we recognized the support of others which included our priest, the funeral director, nurses at the hospital, our pediatrician, the surgeon, and many others. My dear friend, Peggy, from college, came to our house and took over when we needed her. She was a godsend. My husband, Joe, and I were barely functioning."

**Joan**: "Ryan's fiancée and my older son were there for me, but I was numb after dealing with the shock of Ryan's overdose. The police did not make it any easier with their questions."

**Joan** added, "I appreciate my life and have two other adult children. Plus, my extended family is close; we are there for each other in good times and in bad times. As a family, we have had our share of losses. At my age, you can't escape it."

**Carla**: "The shock of the plane crash and the death of Cassandra and her friend were unimaginable. When we arrived at the site of the accident, we were greeted by college administrators and airfield personnel. Everyone tuned in to our vulnerability and showered us with understanding, kindness, and support. They realized how hard it was for us under these circumstances. The bad news came out of the blue and shattered our world. We saw some of Cassandra's college friends, and they cried as they offered condolences. It was the worst week of my life, and the emotional upheaval stayed with me for a long time. Family and friends did their utmost to support us with their love."

**Carla** reported, "My compassion and empathy have grown. I was compassionate and empathetic before our tragedy, but I had not walked in the shoes of someone who lost a child. Now, I know loss, grief, bereavement, and coping. Once you have lived it, you are changed because you have a new appreciation for compassion and empathy. I think the loss of a child is the worst experience ever. Also, when something happens so suddenly you have no time to prepare. I felt numb for so long after Cassandra's death."

**Penny** stated, "I am a widow, too, so Joseph's wife looks to me for support and understanding. I am a good listener, and we all have our love and admiration for Joseph in common. I still have two other sons and a daughter and a slew of wonderful grandchildren."

**Colleen** stated, "I've been through death before, but when it's your kid, it is the hardest. He was such a good kid, too. Sometimes I feel like I'll never get over losing Max, but they say that time helps. I think I have a few more years to go. My son, Bob, and his wife, Linda, went to the hospital a lot. Sometimes Linda would drive me and stay with me so that I was never alone at the hospital. They were supportive and caring."

**Ellen** reported, "My relationships with my husband and kids are strong. My family tries to be supportive of one another. I am close to my sister and niece. I see my parents fairly often, but they live in Florida. I have a big extended family. My father was one of 13 kids."

**Ellen** shared, "I have always had great compassion for others. I'm a sensitive person to the needs of others, but I'm also a strong person. After my life experiences so far, I have grown positively. My kids make me strong. My faith makes me strong. I think I am the biggest advocate for my kids. I realize that I am stronger than I thought I was. When you go through difficult life experiences like losing a child, you come out stronger in the long run. Also, you have to keep going for your other kids. Even though you mourn the loss of that baby, you go through the process of healing. The passage of time helps, too. You never forget about the loss, but you manage to go on for your family."

**Ellen** concluded, "I have a strong work ethic. I try to make the world a better place. My husband and I try to instill good values in our kids, and so far, they have turned out to be good kids. I have two in college at present and one in high school."

**Diane** remarked, "Throughout Darren's long illness, people were kind, supportive, attentive, and compassionate. It was a roller-coaster ride for many years. But we always felt cared for by family and friends. Our pediatrician was there for us every step of the way; he was an amazing man. He is in heaven now with Darren."

**Diane** added, "I have always considered myself to be a kind and compassionate person. However, after living these 13 years with Darren, I have more compassion for the families I met in the hospital over the years who were battling different forms of childhood cancer. My heart goes out to them. It is an emotional roller coaster much of the time from appointment to appointment, treatment to treatment. You have so much hope for these families. You pray for them. In times of trouble, many of us turn to religion and our spiritual side for strength."

**Diane** shared, "My view of myself changed over time. In the beginning, I saw myself as a scared little girl and over 13 years I became a warrior against cancer. I was a strong advocate for my son throughout his long ordeal. At the same time, I had to be there for my other children. Darren's illness took its toll on the entire family, and we all grew strength from him. He had a winning attitude and loved life. We had wonderful family vacations that built such great memories. Even though he is in heaven, so much of him is still with us. I matured as a person and as a mother through the challenge of having a child with cancer."

**Diane** concluded, "I still believe that God has a hand in our lives and that He does not send us challenges that we can't handle. I believe in love, helping others, and making the most of our lives in terms of purpose. But I have come to believe that most of us are stronger than we think we are and that sometimes we have to get out of our comfort zone to make a difference. I am much more of an advocate for my family and others than I was 15 or 20 years ago, and I learned this because of Darren. He made me who I am today."

### Theme: Moving On While Still Broken

The participants in the study shared reasons for moving on with their lives while still dealing with heartbreak. For some, life was dictated by work and family responsibilities. Keeping busy was a form of therapy for some of the women. Some mentioned that they needed to work to pay the bills, and others sought distraction. There was fear of depression, unemployment, and preoccupation with loss.

**Amanda**: "It helped me to go back to work as a nurse. A couple of times there would be someone coming into the ER and it would be a child that died. I wanted to help others because of my own experience. I realized that people listen to you more when you share that you had been through a similar experience. People know that you understand their situation."

**Jean**: "What I took away from this sad, devastating experience was many positives. I want to help people in any way that I can. I try to be the best that I can be because of my granddaughter. Her death put me into action with Sisters by Heart and the March of Dimes. I was energized to do something as I was grieving. Being active and engaging in meaningful activities helped me heal."

**Jean** reported, "I recommend that people do something positive to help with the pain. I tell them my story and how it worked for me. I think keeping busy helps, especially if your efforts are directed toward helping others. It reminds you that you are not in this alone. Both the Sisters by Heart organization, which is based in Minneapolis, and the Grandparent Bereavement Group focus on compassion and understanding. It also helps to know that you are not alone; others are going through similar experiences. Each time I knitted a baby hat for Sisters by Heart, it gave me purpose and made me feel that I was helping another family."

**Jean** continued, "I am a better person and a stronger person now. As a healthcare provider in the pediatric and maternity realm, this gave me a clear lens into what parents and grandparents go through with a very sick newborn, a premature baby, and a child with birth defects. This was up close and personal. Also, I was right there through all of it. You want to be strong for the parents, but your heart is breaking, too, as a grandmother."

**Jean** added, "I see myself now as the best version of myself, and I owe this to my granddaughter, Amy. She changed me for the better and made me want to help more than ever. I now teach about grief and have come to know it well." Jean continued, "I have a strong desire to help people in whatever way I can. I look at the positive side of everything. I live in the moment because we don't know how long we will be on this earth. My spirituality grew as a result of this traumatic experience."

**Barbie**: "Although I was shocked to hear about Jack's death, I mobilized quickly because I knew that no one else in the family would be able to make the funeral arrangements and formulate plans for a Mass at the college chapel. Jack had three ex-wives, and his children were young adults and lived in various locations. I knew that I had to be the one to bring everyone together. I was on a mission to get things done and honor Jack's memory."

**Gloria**: "When my twins were in the NICU, I worked in the hospital's academic laboratory. So, I was able to visit them all the time. Eventually, I was able to get help to care for Lara at home and I went back to work. My schedule was somewhat flexible if I needed to take Lara to a doctor's appointment. My co-workers were wonderful to me."

**Janet**: "After my granddaughter Dana's death, I spent time with my daughter Marian, who was very distraught and needed me. It was very difficult to see my child hurting so much after losing her newborn daughter. Going back to teaching nursing was both a blessing and a reminder of what happened because I teach maternity nursing. As time passed, I knew I was getting stronger. Plus, I realized that I could use my real-life experience as a powerful teaching moment."

**Janet** commented, "When I think about this horrible event that occurred some time ago, I feel that I have moved in a positive direction over time. I think I have grown as a person. A sign of posttraumatic growth was the fact that I was eventually able to teach my nursing students about perinatal loss. In the beginning, I simply couldn't do it, and I asked other faculty to do it. But when we were dealing with Covid-19 on top of everything else that goes on during a semester, I was able to finally do it. I felt like I could, and I briefly told the students that it might be a little difficult for me because I lost my newborn granddaughter. But I was able to do it. This was a big step for me. This exemplified posttraumatic growth for me. When I teach about perinatal loss, I have a PowerPoint presentation, and I have pictures of Dana with her parents. I give a nurse's perspective on how to handle a perinatal loss. I feel strength and growth in myself. In the future, I want to work with groups of nurses and other caregivers on how to be helpful and sensitive in dealing with perinatal loss."

**Janet** added, "I know I have an increased sense of compassion after experiencing this loss. I've always been a 'volunteer-type' of person, helping in the community, and finding ways to give back to my community. I have donated to the food pantry, women's shelter, and soup kitchen. I like to act and do things for people. For example, I make Valentine's gift bags for the kids in the Pediatric Intensive Care Unit at the hospital. I am strong and capable. I think I look at life differently now. I think many people get consumed with things that don't matter that much. I try to focus on what's important by thinking, "Does that matter?" I used to be afraid of death and aging. Now, my outlook has changed for the better. I look at the bigger picture and have a greater appreciation of life. Life is short, and you must stop and appreciate what is around you. For example, I live in the mountains; it's a rural area. I have a greater awareness of nature, like seeing more foxes and birds, and deer in my yard. I refer to them as 'the resident deer' because I see the same ones often. I seem to notice things around me more than I did."

**Janet** added, "It is weird when I look at the timeline of my life because I realize that I have had a lot of losses. Each loss taught me something. I recognize that loss happens. I realize that I am human, and this brings me thoughts of Dana. I acknowledge my sadness. I remind myself of the beauty in this world. I also realize that every human will experience some trauma in their lifetime. We must draw on our experiences and basically 'Let life happen.' I think I have a good outlook on life and a good philosophy of life. My experiences have made me who I am. Lately, meditation and music help me."

**Janet** concluded, "My therapist has pointed out to me that she thinks I have had growth. I have always been a very positive person and even when I am feeling sad, I am not negative. I believe that Dana's short life had a purpose."

**Susan**: "I had to move on for the sake of my three remaining kids. They were all younger than Brianne. I wanted to make sure they were all okay mentally after their older sister's suicide. The kids were confused, bewildered, and felt lost. They needed some stability in their lives, and my husband and I tried to provide as much of that as possible under the circumstances. We learned a great deal from going through this experience. We were better informed about a host of mental health problems after going through this heartbreaking tragedy."

**Susan** added, "I try to be optimistic and live more in the moment, not taking anything for granted. I have educated myself on depression, anxiety, suicide, and things that compromise a person's judgment. I try to be more proactive and educated in raising my children. Bad things can happen to good kids. We tell our kids that it is okay to ask for help. We want them to ask for help whenever they need it."

**Susan** continued, "Eventually, I started to have some growth experiences. I started to have a greater appreciation of life, saw new possibilities through my other children, and had improved relationships with my sisters, brothers, and extended family. People were there for me, being so kind and consoling. I prayed more than usual, and a very religious friend was especially supportive and helped me to realize my spirituality. This helped me forgive myself and stop blaming myself for something that I couldn't control."

**Penny**: "I moved on with my life and made a concerted effort to have a positive and active presence in my son's family. My grandchildren and their mother include me in almost everything. We were always close, but this was a new normal."

**Carla**: "Everyone has their way of coping with tragedy and loss. To be honest, I was in slow motion for a long time, especially for the first year after the airplane accident. When our younger daughter was actively engaged on the playing field or in the gym, she almost seemed normal. But academic subjects took a hard hit with concentration problems, lack of interest, and such sadness about losing her sister. I would cry every day whether I was grocery shopping, driving, talking on the phone, or walking the dog. It was as if I was in this sad trance or altered state of being. I try to be the person Cassandra would want me to be." Carla remarked, "I had to go through the motions of life for my younger daughter and husband. Death is so final even though I have wonderful memories of our family, the four of us. We had great vacations, exciting trips, and so much fun together. I used to think of myself as happy, optimistic, and fun-loving."

**Carla** added, "I believe in not putting things off and living more in the moment. In other words, take that trip, read that book, buy that dress, etc. I also believe that God has been with me through this ordeal and that He has given me the strength to go on."

**Carla** continued, "Surprisingly, I have had some signs of growth after trauma with my appreciation for my family, friends, neighbors, and church. Everyone has been so kind to us. Prayer and therapy have also helped. I have my younger daughter and husband who keep me going. I have a purpose in my life. I have grown closer to my extended family. I think of Cassandra every day and how much I miss her. My heart is broken, but I must go on." Carla added, "I have always been an optimistic and happy person, but losing Cassandra blew me out of the water. I don't know what I would have done without the love and support I received. The people at church were awesome."

**Chantelle**: "After Mark died, I quit smoking. I have smoked since I was a teenager. I tried to set an example for my sons because they smoke and drink beer every day. I want our family to be more health conscious."

**Chantelle** reflected, "I am a pretty strong person. I have had to put up with a lot of different things in my life. My life has been difficult. I think if Mark had behaved differently the outcome would have been different. He had many problems as a child, which continued into adulthood. He resisted advice from everyone who tried to help him. I didn't feel guilty about asking him to leave because I was worried about the other children. It wasn't something I wanted to do, but it was something I had to do under the circumstances. I did the best that I could do. It was really hard. You know, it is very hard when your kid doesn't listen to you or the doctors or the police. It broke my heart, but I had to think of the younger kids at home. I think I have grown stronger with each hurdle thrown at me, or maybe I have just become tougher. Maybe I am just weary of the losses and worries I have experienced in my life. But sometimes I can still laugh about something with a friend. I try not to be all 'doom and gloom.' I laugh about some of the crazy things I see on TV about Donald Trump. I still have a sense of humor. Life can be funny, too."

**Chantelle** continued, "I am close to my two sons. One lives with me, and the other is nearby. I have a few friends that I see. I try to take every day as it comes. Everyone has problems to deal with. Life is not easy. There are good days and bad days. I think Covid-19 worries all of us. I think I have compassion for others. I had compassion for Mark, but I also had frustration with him because he would not follow the doctor's advice and quit smoking to get a kidney transplant. Who knows, maybe he would have been able to turn his life around if he was able to get a new kidney. But he was the one who was unwilling to quit smoking. He chose cigarettes over life."

**Chantelle** concluded, "I have always tried to do the best I can for my family. I think I am a 'survivor.' I think most mothers simply carry on when tragedy strikes if they have kids. Most of the time they don't have a choice unless they have a lot of help from relatives or friends. I never had very much help. When a friend does something to help me, I appreciate it and I thank them. I think that I became a stronger person because I have had to deal with sadness and loss. I have had more than my share of worries over the years. I admit that I am a worrier, which is a bad habit. I don't feel like I have a lot of control over things. I do the best I can for my family. We have never had much money; we just try to get by."

**Colleen**: "I've lost many people in my life, but Max's death hit me the hardest. I think it was because he was such a good person. Due to his heart defect, he was not able to work anymore. I think he was happiest when he worked at a pizza parlor in his twenties and early thirties."

**Ellen**: "Family and work kept me going. Besides having the usual parental responsibilities, I had a business to run. Everyone was understanding and helpful, but at the end of the day, I was 'Mom' at home and 'the Boss' at work."

**Ellen** added, "After Baby Jane died, we have moved in a positive direction as a family; we are close, supportive of each other, and love each other. We acknowledge that Jane was part of our family even though she was only on this earth for a little while. We choose to honor the baby we lost."

**Barbie** recounted, "Once again, I try to find some joy in my life every day. I am grateful and appreciate my life. I believe that we all need to be good to ourselves even if it is only doing one thing a day for ourselves. I have confidence, strength, and integrity and try to be the best person I can be."

### Theme: Never Forgotten, Always in My Heart

All 12 mothers and two grandmothers mentioned their devotion to the child they lost. They said that they would never forget the impact and importance of that child. These sentiments gave testimony to the meaningful nature of the loss.

**Barbie**: "I am so glad that I had that last telephone conversation with Jack. He ended the conversation with 'I love you, Mom.' The next day he was hit by a truck and died."

**Carla**: "My daughter Cassandra is with me every day and holds the pieces of my heart together."

**Gloria**: "When I look at Lara, I wonder what her twin Alice would have been like if she survived."

**Diane**: "My son, Darren, made me the person I am today. He battled cancer for 13 years and never complained or felt sorry for himself. He was a fighter and a great kid."

**Colleen**: "Taking Max off life support was the hardest thing I have ever done."

**Jean**: "It's been eight years since my granddaughter, Amy, died and I still think of her every day."

**Susan**: "I find myself thinking about Brianne and wondering what she would be like as an adult. Questions pop into my mind sometimes, such as 'Would she be a mother?' What career path would she have taken after college? Where would she live?"

**Susan** added, "As the years have passed, we have moved on to a certain extent, but we will never forget Brianne. She was our first child and a smart, beautiful, and amazing person. She had such a bright future ahead of her."

**Janet**: "Dana meant so much to my daughter, Marian, and also to me. We both took on new roles with her birth. Marian became a mother, and I became a grandmother. Those were milestones for us."

**Amanda**: "I can't help but wonder what Carol would be like today. She would be 38 years old. Would she be a nurse like me? Would she be married and have kids?"

**Joan**: "If Ryan had not died of an accidental overdose, he would have married his fiancée. I wonder if they would have had kids. What would their life be like?"

**Ellen**: "My husband, our kids, and I celebrate Jane's birthday every year even though she died soon after birth. It is our way to honor her. Some of my extended family think it's weird, but my immediate family embraces it. It was 15 years ago."

**Carla**: "When I think of what could have been, it makes me sad. Yet, I am grateful for having Cassandra in my life. Memories of her stay with me and are joyful. She is in my heart forever."

### Theme: Holding My Loved Ones Close

Participants in the study attempted to put their loss in perspective by appreciating their remaining family members. Sometimes a death causes people to count their blessings and view others with gratitude and thankfulness. A sudden loss can act as a wake-up call. Often it makes them take stock of their situation and identify who and what is helpful and who and what can be discarded. Frequently, loss leads to the identification of what is significant in life.

Participants found their unique ways of mourning, grieving, and coping. They had their ways of honoring and remembering the one they lost. They found meaning in the experience surrounding the child's death and chose to celebrate their life even if it was brief. The participants held onto memories and tried to view their own lives through a positive lens, which helped to facilitate posttraumatic growth.

**Jean**: "I saw myself as an advocate for my granddaughter and her parents when she was in the NICU."

**Gloria**: "My philosophy of life is that I try to look on the bright side, and my glass is always half full. I believe in new possibilities, hard work, and the golden rule. I believe in love, empathy, and compassion. I try to enjoy life with my family and friends."

**Ellen**: "I value my family, God, and my religion. My husband and I try to instill good values in our kids, and so far, they have turned out to be good kids."

**Susan**: "Brianne's suicide alerted my husband and me to mental health issues in kids. Parents need to be vigilant in observing their kids, and they need to ask the right questions if there are any signs of something being amiss."

**Carla**: "With one remaining child, I must be careful not to smother her with worry and concern and not be so restrictive that I push her away from me. Although I want to protect her from harm, I need to remember that she needs her own space. On the other hand, I don't want to become overindulgent and lax in discipline. I hold Bernadette and my husband close."

**Diane**: "In some ways, I feel that I often gave Darren more attention because he was sick. I need to be there for my girls more than ever. Now, I try to make them both feel special. I like to bake with them, take them shopping, and help them in any way that I can. We enjoy each other's company."

**Janet**: "My daughter Marian has had a tough time dealing with Dana's death. She acted appropriately as soon as she sensed the baby was having health problems. We did everything we could to save Dana. I continue to be there for Marian. We are closer than ever, and we realize that we need each other. I am also close to my two other daughters and my husband. As a family, we try to be there for each other. If Dana had lived, she would be surrounded by loving and caring people."

**Colleen:** "Max was the second youngest out of four boys. They were all young adults when Max died. They all knew about his heart defect and urged him to go to the hospital when his feet became so swollen that he could not wear shoes. We were all scared, including Max. Yet, he was never one to complain. My boys were all wonderful in their own ways."

The aforementioned themes were presented through the lens of PTG, focusing on the death of a child. The themes captured the essence of women's experiences as mothers

Table 4.1 Women Who Lost Children Demographics

| Name | Family Role | Child's Name | Age of Child at Death | Cause of Child's Death |
|---|---|---|---|---|
| Amanda | Mother | Carol | 3 years old | Gastric volvulus, toxic megacolon |
| Susan | Mother | Brianne | 19 years old | Suicide by pills |
| Penny | Mother | Joseph | 62 years old | Scuba diving incident—cardiac related |
| Joan | Mother | Ryan | 26 years old | Accidental overdose |
| Janet | Grandmother | Dana | 5 days old | Hepatic necrosis |
| Barbie | Mother | Jack | 44 years old | ? Suicide by being hit by a large truck |
| Carla | Mother | Cassandra | 19 years old | Plane crash |
| Diane | Mother | Darren | 13 years old | Brain cancer |
| Gloria | Mother | Alice | 6 months old | Prematurity, respiratory failure |
| Colleen | Mother | Max | 42 years old | Chronic heart failure |
| Jean | Grandmother | Amy | 1 month old | Hypoplastic left heart & VACTERL syndrome |
| Chantelle | Mother | Mark | 45 years old | Kidney and heart failure |
| Ellen | Mother | Jane | 7 days old | DiGeorge syndrome and heart failure |

and grandmothers. The words of these women gave testimony to each theme. They acknowledged that their lives were changed forever as a result of their heartbreaking loss. As the years passed, many women shared that they saw elements of PTG in themselves. They spoke of lessons learned from the tragedy and new information gleaned about themselves, their support system, and their worldview. They appreciated life and found reasons to go on living such as the blessings of family and friends. While there is no definitive timeline for the development of PTG or any guarantee that people will experience it, there was a sense of hope in the study participants and recognition of various degrees of PTG as outlined by the five domains of the model.

## References

Baskin, T. W., & Enright, R. (2004). Intervention studies on forgiveness: A meta-analysis, *Journal of Counseling and Development, 82*(4), 79–90.

Bogensperger, J., & Lueger-Schuster, B. (2014). Losing a child: Finding meaning in bereavement. *European Journal of Psychotraumatology, 5*, 22910.

Brabant, S., Forsyth, C., & McFarlain, G. (1997). The impact of the death of a child on meaning and purpose in life. *Journal of Personal & Interpersonal Loss, 2*(3), 255–266.

Buchi, S., Mörgeli, H., Schnyder, U., Jenewein, J., Hepp, U., Jina, E., & Sensky, T. (2007). Grief and post-traumatic stress in parents 2–6 years after the death of their extremely premature baby. *Psychotherapy and Psychosomatics, 76*, 106–114.

Calhoun, L. G., Tedeschi, R. G., Cann, A., & Hanks, E. (2010). Positive outcomes following bereavement: Paths to posttraumatic growth. *Psychologica Belgica, 50*, 125–143.

Cook, P., White, D. K., & Ross-Russell, R. I. (2002). Bereavement support following sudden and unexpected death: Guidelines for care. *Archives of Diseases of Children, 87*, 36–38.

Crenshaw, D. A. (2006). An interpersonal neurobiological-informed treatment model for childhood traumatic grief. *Omega: Journal of Death and Dying, 54*(4), 319–335. https://doi.org/10.2190/b115-5526-0u27-4296

Currier, J. M., Neimyer, R. A., & Keesee, N. J. (2010). Sense and significance: A mixed-methods examination of meaning-making after the loss of one's child. *British Journal of Clinical Psychology, 66*(7), 791–812. https://doi.org/10.1002/jclp.20700

Engelkemeyer, S., & Marwit, S. (2008). Post-traumatic growth in bereaved parents. *Journal of Traumatic Stress, 21*(3), 344–346.

Enright, R. D., & Fitzgibbons, R. P. (2014). *Forgiveness therapy: An empirical guide for resolving anger and restoring hope*. APA.

Foot, C., Gilburt, H., Dunn, P., Jabbal, J., Seale, B., Goodrich, J., & Taylor, J. (2014). People in control of their health and care: The state of involvement. http://www.kingsfund.org.uk/sites/files/kf/field/field_publication_file/people-in-control-of-their-own-health-and-care-the-state-of-involvement-november-2014.pdf

Gerrish, N., Steed, L., & Neimeyer, R. (2014). Meaning reconstruction in bereaved mothers: A pilot study using the biographical grid method. *Journal of Constructivist Psychology, 23*(2), 118–142.

Helgeson, V., Reynolds, K., & Tomich, P. (2006). A meta-analytic review of benefit-finding and growth. *Journal of Consulting and Clinical Psychology, 74*(5), 797–816.

Jenewein, J., Moergeli, H., Fauchere, J., Bucher, U., Kraemer, B., Wittman, L., & Buchi, S. (2008). Parent's mental health after the birth of an extremely preterm child: A comparison between bereaved and non-bereaved parents. *Journal of Psychosomatic Obstetrics and Gynaecology, 29*(1), 53–60.

Keesee, N. J., Currier, J. M., & Neimeyer, R. A. (2008). Predictors of grief following the death of one's child: The contribution of finding meaning. *Journal of Clinical Psychology, 64*(10), 1145–1163. https://doi.org/10.1002/jclp.20502

Li, J., Hansen, D., Bo Mortensen, P., & Olsen, J. (2002). Myocardial infarction in patients who lost a child: A nationwide prospective cohort study in Denmark. *American Heart Association*. https://doi.org/10.1161/01.CIR.0000031569.45667.58

Martincekova, L., & Klatt, J. (2017). Mothers' grief, forgiveness, and post-traumatic growth after the loss of a child. *Omega-Journal of Death and Dying, 75*(3), 248–265. https://doi.org/10.1177/0030222816652803

Michael, C., & Cooper, M. (2013). Post-traumatic growth following bereavement: A systematic review of the literature. *Counselling Psychology Review, 28*(4), 18–32.

Moore, M., Cerel, J., & Jobes, D. (2015). Fruits of trauma? Post-traumatic growth among suicide bereaved parents. *Crisis, 36*(4), 241–248.

Neimeyer, R. (2016). Meaning reconstruction in the wake of loss: Evolution of a research program. *Behaviour Change, 33*(2), 65–79.

Neimeyer, R., Klass, D., & Dennis, M. (2014). A social constructionist account of grief: Loss and the narration of meaning. *Death Studies, 38*, 1–14.

Neimeyer, R. A., Burke, L. A., Mackay, M. M., & van Dyke-Stringer, J. G. (2010). Grief therapy and the construction of meaning: From principles to practice. *Journal of Contemporary Psychology: On the Cutting Edge of Modern Developments in Psychotherapy, 40*(2), 73–83. https://doi.org/10.1007/s10879-009-9135-3

Reilly, D., Huws, J., Hastings, R., & Vaughan, F. (2008). "When your child dies you don't belong in that world anymore"—Experience of mothers whose child with an intellectual disability had died. *Journal of Applied Research in Intellectual Disabilities, 21*, 546–560.

Riley, L., LaMontagne, L., Hepworth, J., & Murphy, B. (2007). Parental grief responses and personal growth following the death of a child. *Death Studies, 31*, 277–299.

Rogers, C., Floyd, F., Seltzer, M., & Hong, J. (2008). Long-term effects of the death of a child on parents' adjustment in midlife. *Journal of Family Psychology, 22*(2), 203–211.

Ronel, N., & Lebel, U. (2006). When parents lay their children to rest. *Journal of Social & Personal Relationships, 28*(4), 507–522.

Saka, Y., & Cohen-Louck, K. (2014). From demonization to identification: How parents who lost children in terrorist attacks perceive the attacker. *Journal of Loss and Trauma, 19*(2), 137–154. https://doi.org/1 0.1080/15325024.2012.743323

Tedeschi, R. G., & Calhoun, L. G. (1995). *Trauma and transformation: Growth in the aftermath of suffering*. Sage.

Tedeschi, R. G., & Calhoun, L. G. (1996). The posttraumatic growth inventory: Measuring the positive legacy of trauma. *Journal of Traumatic Stress, 9*(3), 455–471. https://doi.org/10.1007/BF02103658

Tedeschi, R. G., & Calhoun, L. G. (2004). Posttraumatic growth: Conceptual foundations and empirical evidence. *Psychological Inquiry, 15*(1), 1–18. https://doi.org/10.1207/s15327965pli501_01

Wade, N. G., Hoyt, W. T., Kidwell, J. E. M., & Worthington, E. L. Jr. (2014). Efficacy of psychotherapeutic interventions to promote forgiveness: A meta-analysis. *Journal of Consulting and Clinical Psychology, 82*(1), 154–170. https://doi.org/10.1037/a0035268

Waugh, A., Klemle, G. & Slade, P. (2018). Understanding mothers' experiences of positive changes after neonatal death. *European Journal of Psychotraumatology, 9*(1), 1528124. https://doi.org/10.1080/20008198.2018.1528124

Wheeler, I. (2002). Parental bereavement: The crisis of meaning. *Death Studies, 25*, 51–66.

Worden, W. (2008). Grief counseling and grief therapy. In *A handbook for the mental health practitioner* (4th ed.). Springer.

Zetumer, S., Young, I., Shear, M. K., Skritskaya, N., Lebowitz, B., Simon, N., Reynolds, C., Mauro, C., & Zisook, S. (2015). The impact of losing a child on the clinical presentation of complicated grief. *Journal of Affective Disorder, 1*(170), 15–21. https://doi.org/10.1016/j.jad.2014.08.021

# 5

## WOMEN'S EXPERIENCES OF A CLOSE BRUSH WITH DEATH AND POSTTRAUMATIC GROWTH

A close brush with death is when someone survives a serious accident, injury, or illness. A close brush with death can startle one's senses. It can trigger the "fight or flight" mechanism in most people. Surviving a terrorist bombing, an earthquake, a near-drowning, or a host of other narrow escapes from death could result in a person's life choices and opportunities changing by fostering personal growth and positive changes in an individual. Although the event could result in no appreciable changes at all, conversely, it could be a major stumbling block in a person's life. How a person processes and makes sense of their close brush with death can lead to positive psychological changes about what is important and meaningful in life and what is not. According to Wren-Lewis (1994), after a close brush with death, a person sees the world differently. This may come from both letting go of past assumptions as well as building new ones.

The research study described in this chapter focuses on the experiences of women who had a close brush with death by their estimation. Their past traumatic experience is viewed through the lens of posttraumatic growth (PTG), a conceptual framework written about extensively by Tedeschi and Calhoun (1996, 2004). Our subsequent research study on women who had a close brush with death serves to fill a gap in the literature since there is only a scant amount of published studies on a close brush with death when compared to a robust amount of studies on near-death experiences (NDEs). Not everyone who experiences a close brush with death will report an NDE. Near-death experiences are defined as a spectrum of highly specific and detailed memories associated with the traumatic event (Peinkhofer et al., 2019). These are usually described as out-of-body experiences associated with a tunnel and/or white light; the presence of deceased family members, angels, and/or God; and feelings of calm or peace.

### What Does the Research Tell Us?

There is a scant amount of published research about PTG and close brushes with death. Martin and colleagues (2004) in their work have identified three central contributions to psychological growth that can follow a close brush with death: (1) decreased reliance on

DOI: 10.4324/9781003456650-5

generic knowledge structures, (2) increased reliance on personal experience, and (3) a more benign worldview. The basic tenets of these contributions can be seen as results that are highlighted in some studies exploring a close brush with death and the possibility of PTG developing at some point in the future after the traumatic event is processed and meaning is derived from it.

It is noteworthy to mention that context is especially important when we review studies examining a close brush with death, regardless of whether the person had an NDE or not. Every person is an individual, as is the type of traumatic encounter experienced, whether it be an illness, an accident, a physiological complication, a natural disaster, or a wartime event. It is also important to recognize the personality traits of the person, their history with trauma, their support system, and all of the other factors that come into play when a close brush with death occurs.

Most research about PTG in people who have had a close brush with death and/or a near-death experience has been quantitative research. Khanna and Greyson (2015) assessed 251 survivors of a close brush with death using the 21-item Posttraumatic Growth Inventory (PTGI) (Tedeschi & Calhoun, 2004). Results indicated that those participants who reported a near-death experience were associated with higher scores in the spiritual domain of the inventory and that their visions were perceived as spiritual events. Likewise, Royse and Badger (2017) studied 92 survivors of major burns and found that participants who indicated that religion was a major source of strength and comfort had higher scores on the PTGI and the Near-Death Experience Scale (Greyson, 1983) than those who did not report religion as a personally influential factor (Royse & Badger, 2017).

Martin and colleagues (2016) conducted a mixed-methods study of 17 Australian major burn survivors and compared interview data with PTGI (Tedeschi & Calhoun, 2004) results. The findings were similar to the aforementioned studies of other physical trauma survivors; however, the researchers found some barriers to PTG in participants' relationships with others related to guilt burden and visible scarring. Later, Martin and colleagues (2017) studied whether PTG changed over time after a close brush with death in 73 adult burn patients. The researchers used the PTGI (Tedeschi & Calhoun, 2004) to assess the degree of PTG over six months at two-month intervals. Results indicated that PTG and stress were positively correlated and that growth scores diminished as patients' mental health and affect improved and were highest at the midlevel of physical recovery. This finding supports the notion that PTG is linked to adaptation and coping because greater growth is reported with more stress (Martin et al., 2017).

Levy and associates (2020) explored differences in PTG between 35 hospice patients who experienced end-of-life dreams and visions and 35 hospice patients who did not experience this phenomenon. Posttraumatic growth was assessed by using the PTGI (Tedeschi & Calhoun, 2004). The results indicated significant differences between groups in terms of personal strength. Patients with end-of-life dreams and visions had higher scores on all subscales of the PTGI as well as overall PTG compared to non-dreaming patients. These researchers suggested that dreams and visions at the end of life affect PTG in dying individuals in hospice care (Levy et al., 2020).

The aforementioned research (Khanna & Greyson, 2015; Levy et al., 2020; Martin et al., 2016, 2017; Royse & Badger, 2017) largely reported that people who experienced a near-death experience had higher posttraumatic growth (Tedeschi & Calhoun, 2004) scores than those who did not report a near-death experience. The PTG model domains that usually had the highest scores in these studies were spiritual growth and personal strength, and as stress diminished, so, too, did posttraumatic growth.

Several qualitative studies explored the phenomenon of PTG in other populations, such as individuals with cancer, survivors of a traumatic birth experience, and survivors of intimate partner violence. Oh and colleagues (2021) conducted a cross-sectional study with 148 ovarian cancer outpatients at an urban cancer center. The findings indicated that coping and spiritual beliefs were powerful factors that positively influenced PTG. Similarly, Zhai and colleagues (2019) and Mehrabi and colleagues (2015) studied posttraumatic growth in women with breast cancer. Zhai and colleagues (2019) found four manifestations of PTG that were congruent with four of the five posttraumatic growth model domains identified by Tedeschi and Calhoun (2004). Likewise, Mehrabi and colleagues (2015) equated their findings in a phenomenological study of PTG in 15 Iranian women with breast cancer as consistent with the domains of appreciation of life, spirituality, personal strength, and effective interactions with others as defined in Tedeschi and Calhoun's (2004) PTG model. These two studies about women with breast cancer (Mehrabi et al., 2015; Zhai et al., 2019) illustrate the relevance of the PTG model and its domains as identified by Tedeschi and Calhoun (2004).

Bryngeirsdottir and Halldorsdottir (2022) conducted a phenomenological study with 22 survivors of intimate partner violence. The overarching theme was "I'm a winner, not a victim," and participants credited their positive attitude and personal strength with helping to experience PTG in various domains of Tedeschi and Calhoun's (2004) PTG model. Finally, Beck and Watson (2016) studied an international group of 15 women who reported surviving a traumatic birth in their qualitative descriptive study. The four themes that emerged from data analysis consistently supported four of the five domains of Tedeschi and Calhoun's (1995, 1996, 2004) posttraumatic growth model.

The aforementioned quantitative (Khanna & Greyson, 2015; Levy et al., 2020; Martin et al., 2016, 2017; Royse & Badger, 2017) and qualitative studies (Beck & Watson, 2016; Bryngeirsdottir & Halldorsdottir, 2022; Mehrabi et al., 2015; Zhai et al., 2019) significantly contribute to the literature on PTG and offer consistent support to Tedeschi and Calhoun's (1995, 2004) PTG model. Our current study specifically examines women survivors who describe a close brush with death.

## Our Study Themes

Seven themes emerged from our in-depth interviews with these women. These themes included (1) when trauma happens; (2) the will to survive; (3) support: I'm not alone; (4) a second chance at life; (5) healing and recovery: I'm stronger than I thought I would be; (6) putting the pieces of my life back together; and (7) near-death experiences: Some women had them. The following includes these women's stories in relation to the seven themes.

## Our Study Methods

We studied the experiences of 12 women who reported a close brush with death experience. As in our previous studies about widows and women who lost children, study participants for the current study were recruited through purposive and snowball sampling techniques with our nursing network of colleagues from universities, clinical practice, and professional nursing organizations. We contacted colleagues through email or telephone and acquainted them with our research topic and inclusion criteria for potential participants. Colleagues referred potential participants who met the inclusion criteria and were interested in participating in the study. Their contact information was given to the researchers. An informational letter explaining the study, a demographic sheet, and a consent form were mailed to each potential participant in a self-addressed stamped envelope. After the signed consent form and completed demographic sheet were received, an in-person or telephone interview was scheduled depending on the participant's availability, geographical distance, and Covid restrictions. Again, we limited our sample selection to women who had undergone a close brush with death at least five years before their interviews. We believed that a five-year hiatus was necessary for these women to adjust to their close brush with death experience.

## Theme: When Trauma Happens

### Claudia

"I got very sick in 2015; it was February. I was at a job that I hated. I ate lunch and was okay. I looked at the clock and said to myself, 'I have had a very funny headache all week.' Then, I started to feel really sick. All week I kept noticing a rash on my back and when I touched it, it felt like my back was on fire. So, those were my two symptoms, the headache and the rash."

"I felt sick so I packed up my stuff and left work. I told them that I was sick and had to go home. By the time I got to the car, I felt even sicker. I called one of my kids. Charlene lived in Delaware and I called her because I knew she would be at home. I asked her if I could mix Tylenol with Ibuprofen, and she didn't know. So, she told me to call Sarah, another one of my daughters who was a nurse. Sarah had trouble understanding me because my teeth were chattering so much. At times I was burning up with a fever and at other times I'd be having chills. I got home and told my son and daughter-in-law who were living with me that I was sick and had to go to bed."

"I don't remember much because I was so sick, but I do remember sitting on the bathroom floor throwing up at night. In the morning my son asked me if I was okay, and he told me that he would keep checking in on me. He had to take his daughter to dancing lessons. Then, both Charlene and Sarah called me to check in and said, 'You have to go to the doctor.' I said okay. I remember thinking, 'I think I need to go to the hospital so I'd better take a shower.' That was such a woman thing."

"My son brought me some Gatorade. He found me in a fetal position at the bottom of the bed and told me that my lips were blue. My daughter-in-law, Maria, had come home and she looked horrified. She later told me that I looked like my father right before he died. I was with both my mother and my father when they died. The next thing I remember was that my son, Matt, asked me if he was driving fast enough to the hospital. I was out of it, and I felt as if I was up somewhere looking down at him. Eventually, I went to a therapist who explained what was happening to my brain with the high fever and delirium. At the hospital, they put me in a wheelchair. So, I'm in the emergency room and they told Matt to leave, so he went outside to call his sister Charlene in Delaware. I remember telling Matt that if I got really bad, they should bring me up to Boston."

"The next thing I remember was being wheeled into the ICU. I was out of it, but I remember looking around they were moving me to bed #7 and I thought that was the room where my father died. They said that they needed to intubate me, and I remember thinking that this was my biggest fear because I gag very easily. I remember not wanting them to do it. Matt was with me when they did it. He said I was struggling, and they had to give me some medicine to calm me down so I wouldn't struggle so much. Matt told me that they needed to do it because I couldn't breathe and that I had agreed to it. I don't remember."

"From here on out, I don't remember anything until I woke up in Boston. I think I was admitted to the Community Hospital on Thursday, and they drove me up to Boston on Saturday night. Matt said they told him that they couldn't handle my case at the Community Hospital. A nurse said to my kids, 'I could lose my job for this, but I have worked in hospitals in Boston and they can do more for your mother there, so get your mother up to Boston.'"

"My kidneys stopped functioning, and I had a heart attack. My liver was failing. My lungs were a mess. They said it was septic shock brought on by pneumococcal pneumonia. They started me on antibiotics and tried to put a port in my leg. Later after I recovered from all of this, I ended up losing my leg below the knee."

"I was in the ICU in Boston, and it was a cold, snowy night. My daughters, Charlene and Sarah, were following my ambulance and got into a car accident. Of course, I didn't know any of this because I was out of it. Sarah was driving, and she was pregnant. These drunk kids hit them, and the car was totaled but they didn't get hurt. They spun around, and the car went into a guardrail. Charlene called 911, and the police came. They said, 'We don't know how you got this car off the road because the tire is shredded, and the axle is broken in half.' Charlene went with the police officer, and Sarah had to go in an ambulance as a precaution because she was pregnant, but she was fine. The police got the guys, too, because they had pulled over down the road. The weather was bad. The guys were drunk, and their car was damaged. The police got them. The driver passed the drunk test."

"I don't remember when I came out of the induced coma. They didn't know if I was going to live. They prepared the kids. They were wonderful to the girls. They let them sleep in the hospital where the doctors sleep for the first night. Then they got them an apartment across the street for $10 a night that they use for patients who are getting treatments. The girls stayed there for a week."

"They did everything they could to save my leg, too. So, I woke up about six or seven days later. The girls kept saying, 'You're in Boston' and they kept talking to me till I opened my eyes. I had the tube down my throat so I couldn't talk. My kids were wonderful, so wonderful."

"One particular night was amazing. One nurse worked with me to breathe with the tube; he was great because I hated the tube. My mind played tricks on me: I saw a helicopter flying over my head, I saw kids' toys, and my car came to visit me."

"This one doctor came in to visit me. Previously, there were these two interns nearby talking about me and saying that I was going to have to lose my leg. I knew it was a possibility, and I wasn't that freaked out because I was so happy to be alive. That doctor told the interns to get out and was angry with them. I acted like I didn't hear anything. Later, my daughters and niece were visiting me, and I mouthed the words to them, 'I am not worried about my leg. I am nervous but I am not freaked out. I am so thankful to be alive.' They all said, 'Don't worry about anything, we're all in this together.' Then, we all prayed together."

"I had the worst nightmare of my entire life, ever, ever, ever. I was in Plymouth, and everything was blowing up around me. I love Plymouth where I live. People were blowing up and animals were freezing dead. I was worried that little kids would be hurt or killed. I was running up and down the streets of Plymouth. I thought, 'I have to call my brother, John, but I couldn't find his phone number. I knew it was in my car, but I couldn't find my car.' I thought, 'I'll go in that store and use their phone, but I don't remember his number. What am I going to do?' Then, I heard God's voice. He said, 'You're calling the wrong person.' You know it's like when we're sick and we call the doctor, but we should talk with God first. We should say a prayer first. Then, I started crying, but it was good tears. All of a sudden, I felt something from the top of my head to the bottom of my toes. It was His peace. I looked at the clock and it was 3:00 AM and I said to myself, 'It's all gonna be fine.' I felt such peace with everything. I will trust God no matter what. That's when I get emotional."

"The next morning, they talked about losing my leg and they seemed surprised that I was okay with it. I knew God had a plan for me. I said, 'I'm good, I'm okay with it.' Nothing scared me. I heard them say you're not out of the woods. But nothing scared me. I knew everything would be okay. My life was in God's hands. If I died it would have meant that it was my time."

"They took the tube out of my throat on Valentine's Day. The infectious disease team came in and asked me about the rash I had on my back when I was first admitted to the hospital. They said you didn't have a blood test for bacterial spinal meningitis, but you've had every symptom, so we know you had it. They said we have never seen a blood infection so severe that anyone has survived. I said, 'I know it was a miracle because a lot of people have been praying to God for me.' The three of them said there is no other explanation. The team said, 'What you had was the perfect storm: pneumococcal pneumonia, bacterial spinal meningitis, and RSV, which is a virus. It all came together, and you shouldn't have lived but you did."

"They had put me on dialysis 24/7 for several days and it worked. My lungs also came back. Now I have a few reminders. I had a below-the-knee amputation, but they thought I was too happy, or too positive. They sent someone to talk to me because they thought I was in denial. I said, 'God spared my life and I'll walk again even though I lost my leg.' The counselor said, 'You are not acting normal, you will have delayed grief.' I said, 'I'm not sad, I'm grateful.' She suggested that I have a memorial service for my leg, and I said, 'That's the most ridiculous thing I've ever heard in my life' and I laughed."

"It's been a long road, but I have a wonderful bionic leg. It was a lot of work with physical therapy at McAuley Rehab. They are amazing there. I have a hydraulic ankle, which is top of the line, a $15,000 leg. I go to a support group for people who have lost limbs, and what I love is that they tell you what to do if you are traveling or for exercise. It's informative and helpful because life goes on. I don't call it a stump; I call it my leg."

"I have some physical problems resulting from the septic shock. For example, my hearing has been affected. Eventually, I'll need hearing aids, and I sometimes have ringing in my ears, but I've gotten used to it. My sense of smell is coming back. I had a panic attack in the shower because I had some clumps of hair fall out. I read later that this happens around the three-month mark after septic shock. I lost about a third of my hair and I had bald spots, but my hairdresser is very good at covering them up. This is not a problem now; my hair is okay. For a while, my sense of taste was affected, and everything tasted horrible, but my sense of taste finally came back. My platelets went crazy, so they sent me to a hematologist. I have something very rare called myeloproliferative essential thrombocytosis neoplasia. I could end up with leukemia in the future. But things are looking good with my blood levels, and I'm down to four pills a day from 14. This is a reminder of God's goodness."

### Tara

"I was seven years old. There was a fire in the house, and I was burned. It was Christmas Eve. I was then hospitalized and what I remember of that was that I went into a coma for about three weeks. From what I was told, I was not expected to live. I remember waking up out of the coma and then going back again. I think I did this on and off. I was in the hospital for eight months, and the burns were horrific. The pain was worse when they changed the dressings, and again, it was horrific. I remember screaming, and I was at such a young age."

"When I came home, I was home-schooled for a while because I was not well enough to go to school. I eventually went back to school. They kept me in the same class and promoted me. This was the most difficult time to be with my peers. I was a child model before this traumatic event. I was a child model since 18 months of age. I did TV commercials, runway modeling, magazines, and newspapers, and I was in entertainment as far as singing. My whole life changed as a result of this event of being burned."

"The surgeries after this were approximately every six months up until I was around 18 years of age. There was a lot of reconstruction. I had 26 surgeries in total. I had one of my late surgeries done when I was 30 years of age, and they did a z-plasty because my neck was in such a position that it almost rested on my chest. I had a lot of reconstructive work done over the years."

"I think the most difficult part of this entire ordeal was transitioning back into my life because almost everything had changed. After an event like that, your life changes. I have to say that I had very good support from my parents. They were unbelievable, and I have to say that I was truly BLESSED. They helped me with everything I was going through."

"I have an older sister, three years older than me. My tragic event affected everyone. My sister was the one who tutored me with homeschooling. Before going back, I was ahead of the class. You know children can be very cruel and I must say that was the most difficult part of going back to school. Not being accepted hurt me. Eventually, I did form some close friendships. But it was the starring and ridiculing that bothered me. For example, some kids called me, 'The Bride of Frankenstein.' This was something that occurred when I went back to school."

"Then, in high school, there was a teacher who didn't want to teach me because of the way I looked, and she thought I was stupid and dumb. It was my mother who went to the school and talked with the person and found out how she felt about me. So, I grew up with the feeling that I would never amount to anything in life. Of course, this was not according to my parents but when you think of a teacher feeling that way. It was very difficult."

"I think that I developed empathy after going through what I had gone through. With this came the idea of becoming a nurse. I knew I could say to patients and families, 'I know what you are feeling because I've been through it.' My experience gave me the credibility to help others. I could relate to the patients' experience. I had been through a lengthy hospitalization and many, many surgeries."

"The physical pain, the emotional pain, those feelings are there. I had a sense of empathy for others even if their traumatic events were different than mine. Their situations were also within the realm of injury, disfigurement, and pain. I can say to others, I understand."

"I went on to make something of my life. Looking back, I can say that when I was a child and through the many surgeries, I could tell how people in healthcare felt about me as a patient as soon they came through my doorway and looked at me. I could tell by their non-verbal expression and their behavior. You become very sensitive to it. I remember how I was treated by healthcare providers. For example, I remember vividly a situation with a physician during my eight-month hospitalization. He was a resident and had my mother up against a wall and he was yelling at her because she wanted to know what my temperature was. This was because occasionally I would run temperatures of 104 degrees F or 105 degrees F. This man behaved very poorly toward my mother. I don't know what his problem was, but I remember crying as a result of the way he acted. All my mother did was ask about my temperature because she cared about me. I was her child. Then, he turned to me ignoring my mother, and said, 'Why aren't you eating?'"

"Conversely, the reconstructive plastic surgeon I had was wonderful. He followed me through all my years of care and then retired. I had great continuity of care and a great rapport with this MD. I had a close bond with him, and I trusted him. When I was 30, I had surgery with someone else who was recommended, and everything turned out fine."

### Bambi

"I was in the hospital, and this was a 57-day hospitalization. My pacemaker had been removed as a result of having an infection of the tricuspid valve of my heart and also an infection on one of the leads to the pacemaker. So, I was without the device which would help my heart function and I was heavily monitored and in the cardiac intensive care unit."

"I was without the pacemaker for four weeks while the infection was being resolved with medication, and each of those four weeks I had a TEE, a transesophageal endoscopy, where they take you to a separate facility within the hospital where they do these kinds of procedures. They put a tube in your mouth that goes down the esophagus, and once the tube reaches a certain level it can visualize what is going on with your heart. This is done under anesthesia. They put a block in your mouth to maintain the integrity of your lips and teeth. They use Propofol, and there is an anesthesiologist and a cardiologist in the room who sits at the computer to see the visualization. So, I had four of these, one week apart because they didn't want to put another pacemaker in if there was any infection left. Then, they finally put in another pacemaker and put it on the opposite side. The pacemaker I have now is on the right side of my chest."

### Rose

"I was a flight nurse in the US Air Force. I was the medical crew director on the Air Force C-5 aircraft on an air evac flight for Operation Babylift that crashed in Saigon, South Vietnam on April 4, 1975. The mission was that we were going to be taking about 300 people out of Vietnam, and most were children under the age of two. Saigon was falling into the hands of the North Vietnamese forces, so we needed to get people out quickly. There was a cadre of women who were going to be accompanying the children, and most were embassy secretaries, dependents of military and embassy personnel that had agreed to help with the children in flight. Our medical crew was three flight nurses and six aero-medical technicians."

"The C-5 aircraft has two levels for passengers and cargo. Once we had the top level of the plane filled, we put older children downstairs on the interior sides of the plane, securing them with cargo straps, blankets, or anything we could find. We had to put some of the attendants on the floor sitting with infants in cardboard bassinets. I assigned the other flight nurses and aeromedical technicians to provide care for the children on either the top-level troop compartment or the lower level of the C-5. We took off and were climbing to altitude over the South China Sea. All of a sudden, we had a rapid decompression. The plane's back 'clamshell' doors had blown out. When I looked down from the grating on the top level of the plane, I could see the South China Sea out the back of the plane. There was no way to get down to the lower compartment to check on people; the ladder connecting the upper and lower compartments was gone, so I had to stay in the troop compartment. I could not tell what was going on downstairs because communication was cut. I could see how damaged the aircraft was with the back clamshell doors missing, so we knew we were going to have a crash landing."

"Once we had the rapid decompression the aircraft commander turned the plane around and headed back to Tan Son Nhut Air Base (Saigon). My focus was on emergency procedures and trying to keep everybody safe. We went through the upper compartment, resecured the babies, and did everything we could to make sure they were secure. When we finally did that and I had designated who would do what, we then hit the ground. I sat on the floor facing forward so I could see what was happening with the babies. There were no windows so you couldn't see anything. The first impact wasn't bad. We crashed two or three miles short of the airport. It wasn't a bad impact that I felt, but on the top level, you are almost six stories above the ground. We bounced airborne over the Saigon River and then we crashed again, but this time it was a much, much more violent hit. Unbeknownst to us at the time, we sheared off the whole bottom level of the aircraft. We coasted along in the rice paddies. The flight deck (cockpit) separated from the aircraft. I was thrown against a wall. There was one moment when I thought, 'I am going to live through this.' I think before that moment we all thought that we wouldn't make it. It all happened so fast. It was only 20 minutes from the rapid decompression till we crashed. A lot happened in those 20 minutes."

"When we crashed, everybody except the charge medical technician in the lower compartment died. Upstairs we lost one adult attendant and one of the babies. I had some injuries but didn't realize it because of the adrenaline rush. I looked out and saw the flight deck about a 90-degree angle away from us. It was upside down, and I thought they must have all gotten killed. But, lo and behold they were all fine. They climbed out of the flight deck and came running over to help. There were 340 people on the plane, and slightly more than half survived. Three of our medical crew were killed, one flight nurse and two aeromedical technicians. The nurse and one technician were from my squadron, which made it very difficult for me."

### Julie

"About seven years ago, I was walking home from work. I'm an usher in the theater district in NYC. The show got out and it was around 11 PM. I had almost reached my apartment when I was mugged. A guy jumped me from behind. He came out of nowhere. He kept yanking at my purse, which was across my body with a long strap. I didn't want to give it up because it had my keys, credit cards, cell phone, money, make-up, and my paycheck. I was walking to the ATM near the corner of my street to deposit the check before going home."

"He was a big man and also tall. He towered over me. He hit me in the face and head and threw me to the ground. No one was around. I tried to scream, but he put his gloved hand over my mouth. He wrestled with me as I became tangled with the strap of my purse. He finally got the purse and belted me again in the face. I was in a state of shock, and I knew my face was bleeding. I had lived in NYC for several years, and nothing like this had ever happened to me. Sometimes my friends and I would go clubbing into the wee hours of the morning, and we never had a bad experience. I remember lying on the sidewalk crying. I couldn't call 911 because my cell phone was in my purse. Finally, a couple came along and helped me up and called 911. The police and an ambulance arrived very quickly. They took me to the hospital. I had a black eye, facial bruises, a cut near my eyebrow, and a very swollen and bruised lip. I was a mess. It had all happened so fast."

"They took care of me in the ER and sent me for a CAT scan of my head. I needed stitches for the cut near my eyebrow. The police questioned me, and the ER doctor admitted me to stay overnight in the hospital. I was in no condition to go back to my apartment. My two girlfriends with whom I shared the apartment came to get me in the morning. They took turns that week staying home with me. There was no way I could work. I was a nervous wreck, and I looked horrible. It was such an awful experience. It was so frightening. I was overwhelmed with fear, and the whole experience scared my girlfriends, too. They knew if it happened to me; it could happen to them. We all swore that we were going to buy Mace or pepper spray."

### Samantha

"In 2013, I was an ICU nurse and I had a lot going on. I had another business with a family member. I was more stressed than usual. I was exhausted. I noticed that I started to get a small bald patch on the back of my head. I went to see my primary care provider, and she couldn't find out what was going on. So, I was referred to a dermatologist. By the time I got in to see the doctor, the bald patch had gotten bigger, and the dermatologist attributed it to stress and told me to do yoga. I knew that it was not normal for someone's hair to fall out and I thought 'This is crazy,' but I did do yoga. Then, I went to see a different dermatologist and finally a specialist at Yale. By then the hair on the back half of my head was gone. Plus, I just never felt good and wondered if all this was really due to stress."

"They tested me for Lyme disease twice, and the tests were negative. They started me on very high steroids to try to stop my immune system from attacking my hair follicles. Unfortunately, what they did not know was that I did have Lyme disease and that it just was not coming up positive on the normal western blot test. About a month later, I was at a wedding, and I was out on the dance floor dancing. I must have had a BLEB (a small fluid-containing cyst in the lung) because I ended up with spontaneous pneumothorax and I required a chest tube. I had to go emergently in the middle of the night to the ER, and I remember being in so much pain. I was tachycardic, and my heart was in cardiac tamponade. It was bad, they had to release the air on the way into the ER. After that, I got sicker after the chest tube came out. I was home from work for a few weeks, and I'd tried to walk around and I noticed that I couldn't feel my feet and my calves were starting to feel tingling. In general, I just didn't feel good. Then, I ended up having a herniated disc that had to be surgically repaired. In November 2013, I went to a neurosurgeon. He told me how his wife was essentially crippled from tick-borne illnesses, and he said to me, 'You definitely have Lyme.' He said that he was going to do more blood tests for Lyme and send them to a different lab than the previous ones. He said, 'Let's get you treated if the tests come back positive."

"So, I had my back surgery and found out in December 2013 that I did have Lyme disease. It went a year undetected. In that year, he thought that maybe it simmered because I had so much other stress. They call Lyme disease the great imitator. So, it would weaken links in my immune system and take advantage of it. I am predisposed to a bunch of autoimmune stuff. So, that's where the alopecia and neuropathy came from. By the time I got to a Lyme specialist, I probably had gone a year without treatment, not knowing that I had the disease."

"Also, the dermatologist had put me on 60 mg/day of Prednisone for 3–4 months, and then he put me on Cellcept. The steroids exacerbated the Lyme and probably did not help my immune injury. I was on intravenous and by-mouth antibiotics for about a year and a half. In that time frame, I had to quit my job as a bedside nurse because I couldn't be on my feet for a couple of hours at a time. I was also in graduate school at the time and sometimes had to stay home and miss classes but fortunately got through the program."

"By the time my husband and I got married, which was probably about a year after the diagnosis, I had lost all of my hair. I was forced to shave my head. I think the second time I wore a wig was on my wedding day. I also remember being helpless and unable to sleep and in constant pain. We have a two-floor house, and I couldn't sleep in our bed because it was on the second floor. I lived on our couch for several months. Sometimes I would drag myself to the other end of the house. My husband would have to help me put on pants sometimes. Lyme annihilated me. So, I went to another neurologist who diagnosed me with chronic demyelinating neuropathy. With people who have this, something disrupts their immune system and causes it. So, Lyme caused this to happen. For me, my bilateral lower extremities slowly demyelinated and the point that he said was at mid-thigh. He said, 'You are killing your short fiber nerves halfway up your legs already.' At that point, I continued antibiotics for a little while longer and used immunoglobulins IgG IV. I got this weekly. I have done those just until recently in 2021. I was on these IVs for seven years. I was at home and had three home care nurses over time. Up until recently one of my nurses was my mother who at least got to see her grandkids. Also, she was paid to be here, which was great. The beginning part of it was hard because it was just me sitting on a couch. Also, after the IV you don't feel very good because they give you profound dehydration. I have had aseptic meningitis three times. It has not been an easy road."

"Three years ago, I started to go to a dermatologist at Yale, who is a genius. He discovered that in people with autoimmune alopecia, the feedback loops that attack the hair follicles operate through 'A Jack,' so he put me on a 'Jack' inhibitor, which is called Zeljam, and over the last few years after I had my kids, my hair has grown back. It is blocking my immune system from attacking my scalp. I was bald for seven years. It's been a slow process for it to grow back, but he says that I was one of those patients that had an immune system that would refuse to stop attacking my head. He said, 'Your hair is stubborn.' Also, the Zeljam has helped my neuropathy. After being on Zeljam for almost a year, I have full recovery of the nerve endings in my legs. It's been great, but this all has been such a slow process. It is all about having patience, which is hard when you are not feeling good. You are trying to do the things in life that you enjoy such as being married and having kids. All of these things have been a struggle on my end."

"I was 33 when this started, and now I'm 40. It was a big chunk of my life, and those are usually fun years, but they weren't for me until I started feeling better. I had to be approved to get pregnant. My husband and I were married for about a year and four months when they said that we could start trying to have a family, and by God's grace we were pregnant in a month. I went to a maternal–fetal specialist, and they approved me to stay on the IV IgG for the whole time. Both of my babies were fine and very healthy. With my son, I felt amazing. I felt like I could run a marathon. My hair started to grow back in the third trimester. Then with breastfeeding, it all fell out again. A year and a half later I had my daughter, and I felt terrible right from the beginning. I never felt good; everything always hurt. I had sciatica, and I could feel every joint in my body. I found out that I was pregnant the week I graduated with my master's degree. So, I went from thinking I would have a break to going back to work and having my daughter."

"Right now, I feel pretty good. I have to do a lot of self-care with yoga and other stuff. I live on a lumbar roller. But I am so much better than I was. I am mostly recovered. My neurologist told me that I'm the only patient with CIDP that has ever recovered. He said that 40% of patients with CIDP become wheelchair-bound as seniors. He said that I was fortunate to recover enough to enjoy life again and work and have kids."

"When I first got so sick, it was so frustrating because I was this busy person. Nurses are busy-bodies and nosy and like to experience life to the fullest. We are constantly traveling and socializing and working. My mind could do things, but my body couldn't. It was so depressing. It was also difficult being bald in my 30s. It takes some of your femininity away from you. It was especially hurtful because I was a newlywed and so much was taken away from me. It was horrifying and hard on my self-esteem for the first three years."

"My husband was totally on my side the whole time. In the beginning, he would come to all my appointments with me. He was very supportive. I have known my husband for 20 years. When we started dating, we were both looking for a new church. We were both raised Catholic, but we found this wonderful non-denominational church. It was like we were doing this Faith Walk together. That was very helpful for us to rely on God. We knew that we had to put each other first to serve our relationship. The funny thing is that as I evened out and could do more and work a little, he was, 'You are okay and can deal with it, right?' I have heard from other people with chronic illnesses that when they feel better, others assume they can push through, and sometimes you have to remind them that you don't always feel that well. It's like he was so used to hearing my report about how I was feeling that it became commonplace like talking about the weather. He was conditioned to hear about it so much that when I was ill he was like, 'What do you mean that you need to lie on the couch all day?' I had to clarify that 'I can't do this today.' He was so used to me pushing through stuff that he'd say, 'Take the Motrin and you'll feel better.' But that was not always the way it was. I still had limitations. I would tell him that sometimes he needed to hear me out and let me complain to relieve some of the pressure. A key phrase for us in some of our conversations was 'I just need you to listen to me.' He got it, too. He's a great guy!"

"That first year and a half of being sick was lonely, too. A lot of my girlfriends were getting married. My family knew that I was ill, but nobody understood the extent of it.

They would think, 'Oh, wow she's losing her hair, that's creepy.' When you are sick and it's not cancer or surgery it is amazing how quickly people forget to be supportive. There were a lot of long nights, and I would just stay up because I had insomnia. I was grateful for the opportunity to find faith and deal with things and compartmentalize some of that pain. It was also amazing how many specialists wanted to throw opioids at me! Everybody wanted to give me pain meds. I understand how so many people become addicted to heroin. At one point one of the doctors offered me Fentanyl patches and I said, 'No!' He said, 'I know how serious your pain is and I want to help.' I said, 'No!' I knew my pain was a ten out of ten at times, but I said, 'If you put me on that now, you are putting a nail in my coffin because, for the rest of my life, I will need those meds, and I don't want them!' I said, 'I cannot do that to my body!' They would always say, 'Well it's your decision.' Some tried to throw Ativan at me, and I said, 'I don't want this!' As a nurse, it has given me great credibility with patients because I have lived with serious pain without taking opioids. I could also help cancer patients dealing with hair loss. For women, it is one of their biggest fears. I would show them as I flipped some of my wigs off because I didn't use the stuff that helps to hold it on. After all, it is hot and sticky. They could see my bald skin and I'd tell them that they were gonna get through this just like I got through it. I think I helped them. I would say, 'This is not your end-all, and it doesn't have to be.'"

### *Millicent*

"I was having my first baby. I had a normal pregnancy. I was 30 years old and in excellent health. I went into labor two days past my due date. Labor started around 6 AM with my water breaking, and the amniotic fluid was clear. Contractions started about 30 minutes after my water broke. Everything was pretty normal, and my husband Larry and I arrived at the Birth Center around 3 PM. The weather was bad, and an ice storm was predicted, so we left the house earlier than planned. When we arrived the baby's heart rate was in the normal range, and I was doing well breathing through the contractions. I spent a lot of time laboring in the shower at the Birth Center."

"My nurse-midwives Florence and Justine were there to keep a watchful eye on me and the baby. At approximately 9 PM I was ten centimeters dilated and had the urge to push. I was tired but mustered up the energy to push. My entire labor was felt in my back. My husband was good at giving me counterpressure on my back. I did not take any pain medication. I wanted a natural birth with an alert baby entering the world. I pushed on and off for almost four hours in a variety of positions to try to rotate the baby's head. I used a squatting bar, which helped. Right before I gave birth, the contractions were felt in the front because the baby's head had rotated to what they call an OA or occiput anterior position. In other words, the baby came out facing the floor. That's how most babies come out."

"Finally, at 1:08 AM I gave birth to a beautiful healthy baby boy. I remember saying to him as I cradled him in my arms, 'I have been waiting for you all my life.' He was such a handsome little guy, weighing in at 7 pounds and 9 ounces. I had gained 25 pounds during the pretty average pregnancy. My husband and I were overjoyed! We kissed each other and our son, Chandler Matthew. Everything seemed fine for a few minutes, and then all of a sudden, my midwife, Justine, grabbed my arm and started putting in an IV. I asked her what she was doing, and she replied, 'You are bleeding a lot.' My other midwife, Florence, started massaging my abdomen. The problem ended up being that the placenta was not coming out as it is supposed to do within several minutes after the baby is born. Both midwives were very concerned because I guess I was losing a lot of blood. They quickly wrapped me in blankets and put me on a stretcher to go across the street to the hospital. I kept Chandler on my chest the whole time. He was fine, but I was not. Larry helped the midwives push the stretcher across the street. He told me later that he was scared out of his mind that I was going to bleed to death. I don't remember losing consciousness, but I think I drifted in and out. What I remember most was having a terrible headache, probably the worst one I have ever had in my life."

"The obstetrician on call tried to manually remove the placenta, which came out but they were not sure if they had all the pieces of it. I endured all of this without any anesthesia or pain medication. It was very painful, and I remember this was the only time I moaned loudly. We had to wait for an anesthesiologist to arrive at the hospital for the operative procedure known as a D&C. They were giving me a lot of IV fluids, and they were waiting for blood from the blood bank for a transfusion. I did not want to go to sleep with general anesthesia because I wanted to be able to see my baby and also because I was afraid I would never wake up. The doctors listened to me and gave me a spinal instead. It was the middle of the night, so they let Larry sit next to me holding the baby during the surgery. My midwives stayed with me, too. I ended up getting six blood transfusions in total and staying in the hospital for five days. The doctor told me that as pale as I looked when I was hemorrhaging, my husband looked worse. Larry was afraid that he would have to raise Chandler without me. I remember talking to my midwives the next day saying that I was afraid of getting AIDS because they weren't screening the blood yet. I think they started screening blood the next year. I was fortunate that the hospital was in an affluent community with an active blood bank on the premises. There would have been a higher risk of tainted blood if I was at an inner-city hospital."

"After this scary near-death experience, I have great respect for Mother Nature and the birthing process. My nurse-midwives were wonderful and took immediate action. Their backup obstetrician was great, too. I am an example of why women need to give birth in a birth center on hospital grounds and not at home unless they live very close to a hospital. Emergencies can happen to healthy women who have normal labor. A postpartum hemorrhage like mine can come out of the blue. I had no risk factors. I think my uterus was tired of laboring and I had been pushing for a long time to rotate the baby's head. I still consider my birth experience to be a positive one because it was natural without medication, and I received excellent care from the midwives and obstetricians. Also, I could not have weathered the storm of labor without Larry's loving support. He never left my side. Having this baby was a team effort. I thank God every day for Chandler and Larry and our other three children, a total of two boys and two girls. A perfect family!"

### Norma

"I was sick with a gastrointestinal virus. I kept working and even took a few extra shifts because I did not want to be home with my first husband. I ended up with Guillain–Barre syndrome. I was in the hospital for six months. I was paralyzed for six months and was in the intensive care unit. I was on a ventilator for at least four weeks and unable to talk and because of the paralysis I had difficulty communicating anything. Mentally I was with it. Soon, I became more talkative especially when the vent was removed."

Norma related, "My spirituality and belief in God is interesting. I probably didn't go back to the church between being so sick and getting divorced. I started going to church again when I got remarried and when I had kids. Seth and Mitch, my sons, have had a great impact on my life. Mitch especially has made me more spiritual. He is at the university studying theology, philosophy, religions of the world, and spirituality. I also think I became more spiritual when Aaron had prostate cancer. Thankfully he recovered."

### Sarah

"I was in the airport in North Carolina. I was with my granddaughter who was 16 years old. We were going to celebrate her birthday and she had never flown on an airplane before, so I flew down from New Jersey and was going to fly back to New Jersey with her. We were going to do some fun activities for the weekend and maybe go into NYC to see a play or something. This was in 2008. This was the day after Thanksgiving. I had retired from the place I was working. Before I left the airport in New York, I ate a sandwich, and at the North Carolina airport, I started having this pressure in my chest. I thought it was indigestion, which I sometimes get. So, I asked my granddaughter to go over to a store in the airport to get me some Tums and a bottle of water, which she did. So, I drank some water and chewed some Tums, but I didn't feel any better. Then, I started to have this choking sensation in my throat and neck as if someone had their hands around my neck trying to choke me. I started walking toward the gate with my granddaughter and 'the lights went out.' I remember being on the floor in the airport and an EMT was saying my name, 'Sarah, Sarah.' She told me the ambulance was on the way and that they would take care of me. I asked her what happened, and she told me to relax, lie back, and that I would be okay. I must have become unconscious at that point. I remember fading in and out and being in an ambulance. I felt the motion of the ambulance. When I got to the hospital, they rushed me to the cardiac catheterization lab, and they put in a stent. I remember waking up in a hospital bed and the nurse came in and greeted me. She said, 'You were lucky to have the heart attack in an airport where help was readily available.' I started looking around the room and wondered whom she was talking to about a heart attack. I didn't know I had a heart attack."

"Of course, after all of this, I eventually sent for my records being the nosy person I am (laughing). This was probably a month after I was home. The notes said that I coded three times in the ambulance and that they were able to put the stent in within 30 minutes of my arrival at the hospital. Someone told me that the hospital I was at was the only hospital in the country that could stent you in under 30 minutes, so I was fortunate to be there. I was blessed. The admitting note also said, 'Notify the family immediately, this is not good, and I don't expect this patient to survive.'"

### Cecilia

"I was about 14 years old. In the summer months, I would go with friends after catching a bus in the city to a place called Crystal Lake. We would go to this lake to go swimming. I had many swimming experiences because I was a junior lifeguard and I got training at summer camp. One of the girls' mothers came with us, and we were having a great day swimming. We went out to a raft in the middle of the lake. Before going on this trip, I was rushing to pack whatever I needed and I always burn easily, I get a sunburn. So, my mother always said to wear a tee shirt so I wouldn't get burned. So that morning I couldn't find a tee shirt, so I grabbed a sweatshirt instead. So, we went to Crystal Lake."

"So, I was swimming with the sweatshirt on. We went out to this raft and there was no problem, we were laughing and joking. Then, I decided to jump in. When I jumped into the lake, the sweatshirt came over my head and I could not get it to loosen up no matter what I tried. The water was trapped in the sweatshirt, and I could not get the sweatshirt off. I don't think the others knew that this was happening. I certainly knew, and I was becoming very panicked. I understand that panic can immobilize. That's exactly what happened. I then felt a sense of relaxation. In front of me flashed different scenes of my life. And, I know at 13 or 14 you don't have much of a sense of life. I saw my parents, I saw myself, I saw Thanksgiving, and I saw Christmas. These were all like flashes of my life through the years. I guess they were like things that were special to me. Then, all of a sudden, I don't remember anything after that. And, the next thing I know, I'm on the raft, the sweatshirt is off me, and people are working on me. They turned me over, and I remember being struck. I woke up and I was very shaken up; someone said I had nearly drowned. I couldn't believe that because of my ability to swim. I was very shaken up. So, they got a boat and brought me to the shore. There were medics there, the ambulance had come, and they checked me out. They did not take me to the hospital. They let me stay at the lake, but I sat it out for the rest of the day. I was very shaken by the event. I thought nothing more of the situation other than being shaken up. I kept saying in my head, 'You almost died, you almost died.' My friends said, 'You are lucky,' and they gave an account of what had happened. They said they saw my head go under and not come back up. First, one person jumped in, then a second person jumped in, then my friends dragged me out of the water. Then, one man who was there helped, too. The water was pretty deep. It said that the water off the raft was 14 feet deep."

"So, after all this, I just sat on the blanket and relaxed. Someone gave me their tee shirt so I wouldn't get sunburned. I didn't think much about it till time passed. When the time had passed, I thought, well, I had lost an uncle in a plane crash when I was about ten years old. I grew up on a street that had a funeral home, so almost daily I saw crowds of people out on the street grieving. And I thought, why didn't I die? And I had deep spirituality at that time. I was a novena girl; I was at a novena every week handing out pamphlets with a blue cape and skull cap. And I just felt there was a reason. So, I would go to church, and I would look up, and I was very connected to the Blessed Virgin, and I would say 'What do you have for me?' 'Why did you spare me?' I realized I had never told my parents about my near-drowning because I believed that they would never let me go to the lake again."

"At that point, I realized I had to do something meaningful with my life. I always looked around at people, and what were they doing in their lives that was meaningful? So, when I was 16 years old, I went to Polyclinic Hospital to volunteer as a candy striper. Then, for two summers, I went to Bellevue Hospital as a candy striper because I wanted psych nursing, and they sent me to the neurology unit where they had people with traumatic brain injuries. As I spent two summers at Bellevue Hospital, I felt a sense of purpose and meaning. I still think I was spared for that reason; I had a contribution to make. I went into nursing. I also was fleetingly tempted to go into show business. My father would say, 'Stick to nursing, you can try show business later.' He said you need to do something so that you can be independent. I never attempted to do anything but nursing. As I look back, my life was spared to help others."

### Eve

"I was working as a waitress at the time, and I was driving home from work after a long shift. It was around 11 PM. It was winter, and the roads were icy and snowy. I must have hit a patch of black ice or something. My car skidded and spun out of control. It hit a guard rail, flipped over, and went down an embankment. I was knocked unconscious. To be honest, I don't know exactly how long it took them to find me. There were not very many cars on the road because the weather was bad. It was a one-car accident. The police and an ambulance arrived at some point. I only know what I was told while I was in the hospital. Although I was on the main road, it was very dark and there were not very many overhead lights. It was such a miserable night weather-wise that I guess most people were staying home."

"I vaguely remember waking up in the ER or maybe it was the ICU with doctors and nurses telling me that I was in a serious car accident. I was in and out of consciousness and don't remember a whole lot of details. Everything was quite a blur, and it stayed this way for quite a while, maybe days or weeks. When I was a little more 'with it,' they told me that I had sustained a subdural hematoma in my brain, a broken arm, and a broken leg. I also had cuts and bruises scattered all over my body. I was a mess. To make a long story short, I was in the ICU for at least a week, then on another unit in the same hospital, and then I was transferred to a rehab facility."

"I recall visits from my boyfriend and my parents. I was pretty out of it when I was in the ICU. I think I was getting a lot of pain medicine and I was sleeping a lot, too. This accident happened five years ago, and there are still some details that I can't remember. The car accident happened so fast. One minute, I was driving, and the next minute the car was spinning, and the rest I don't recall. I guess I'm lucky to be alive."

### Ivana

"I had two different kinds of cancer. The first was breast cancer and then as I was recovering from the breast cancer, I had acute myelogenous leukemia. I think it was during leukemia that I felt that my life might be over pretty soon because I was told that if I didn't get into the hospital right away and get treated immediately, I wouldn't be there for a week. So, not having a lot of choices at that point, my cousin, who was an oncologist, suggested that I go to the medical center. I went right in through the emergency room and got admitted and they started the treatment the next day. The treatment is to destroy your immune system and destroy all the blood cells. They do that and make you so vulnerable, so they have to put you on antibiotics, antifungals, and antivirals to ward off any infection. It does a number on you. I was really sick and very weak. I could barely pick my head up off the pillow. I didn't know if I was going to make it or not. A couple of times they moved me from a semi-private room to the ICU because I started having high fevers, coughing, and chest pain. I developed pneumonia and they had to treat me for that. Of course, the care in ICU was wonderful. I got through that, but this happened a couple of times. I also in the process developed C-diff (clostridium difficile) and I became dehydrated. I went through that sense of 'I hope I make it, but I'm not sure.'"

"I think the thing that got me through was that I just decided that I wanted to live, it was 2014 when I got leukemia. I was 69, and I just decided that there was so much to live for. I wanted to survive, and I had to maintain this positive sense that I could get through all of this. Thank God I did. The people from work were so nice and sweet. I had everybody praying for me. I think my prayers and those of all these other people got me through this. I remember there was this one guy, whom I didn't see eye to eye with on a lot of things. Well, he had been quite sick a few years before, and he had gone to Lourdes and had gotten this bottle of holy water; well, he gave it to me. And I thought, what a wonderful gesture. So, I felt like I had all these people cheering on the side and my determination got me through. I'm just thankful that I'm here."

## Theme: The Will to Survive

**Claudia**, who survived septic shock syndrome, remarked, "I am strong and I fought to live with God's help. I knew God had a plan for me. He wanted me to go on and do all the things I was doing for others. God saved me; He spared my life. I am so fortunate, and I appreciate my life so much. I am still here to enjoy my children and grandchildren, my friends at church, and all the things I like to do in my community. I am so blessed."

**Tara**, a burn survivor, related, "When you go through suffering, you can either crawl into a little ball and never come out or you realize that the struggle has meaning. I grew from the suffering and the struggle. It was a time of growth for me. My trajectory in life could have been quite different had I not been seriously burned on that Christmas Eve night at age seven. This event occurred, and I made it, and each day I thank God. God knew there was something I could do and do well. He had a plan for me. This is where my spirituality comes in."

**Bambi** survived a serious cardiac infection. She recalled, "I am a fighter and fought to survive. I always felt as though I was a strong person, and this illness reinforced that. I feel even stronger than I was after going through this. I felt strong and independent, and this experience helped me in my perception of self. I went ahead believing that I was a strong person and that I can take on things."

She continued, "I was grateful to have come through the experience, and I think that is associated with the confidence I had in the physicians, the hospital, and the staff. I think of it more as gratitude than trauma. I feel growth as a person and am grateful to have survived that experience. I think it gave me an additional perspective very much akin to when I had cancer of the cervix. I came through that procedure as well. From both health experiences, I felt growth and appreciation for life. I think I have an increased responsibility for what I should do with my life. I wanted to be everything that I can be. I wanted to take responsibility for being the best kind of person I can be both professionally and personally. I also wanted to find some joy in each day and enjoy the rest of my life."

**Rose** survived a plane crash in Vietnam. She related, "I know I am a strong person who appreciates life a great deal and had the will to survive the crash. My view of myself as a strong person was reinforced by this traumatic experience. I am strong and a leader without being pushy or domineering. I am confident, but I am also open to the opinions and advice of others. But it has taken me many years to process all of this. I have always welcomed new possibilities, cared deeply about family and friends, and feel great compassion for others. The people who were killed or seriously injured in the plane crash weighed heavily on my mind for years. It was a horrible disaster, but Operation Babylift was a necessary humanitarian mission. We saved many lives by taking these orphans out of war-torn Vietnam. I have reflected on that day so many times. I feel quite spiritual about it."

**Norma** survived Guillain–Barre syndrome when she was in her mid-20s. She remarked, "I came to realize that I am stronger than I thought I was. When I was sick and on a ventilator, I still had a steadfast determination to survive. I just wasn't going to let my life end when I was so young. I wanted to eventually get married and have a family."

**Cecilia** almost drowned while swimming with friends. Cecilia recalled, "I had a strong will to survive. I fought hard to get untangled from my sweatshirt that had entrapped my arms so I couldn't swim. Luckily, my friends saw my predicament and came to my aid. I had my whole life in front of me. Thank God that this situation didn't turn into a tragedy. I am so grateful to my friends for saving me."

**Ivana** had breast cancer and leukemia. She recalled, "I have been in remission now for seven years from both cancers. My will to survive was strong then, and it continues to be strong now. I have three grandchildren who are all in elementary school and I want to live to see them graduate from college. I watch my diet, go on long walks every day, keep all my doctor's appointments, and do everything I can to lead a healthy life. My kids and my husband are all very supportive. We have a very loving family."

### Theme: Support—I'm Not Alone

**Samantha**, a nurse who had severe Lyme disease, shared, "My faith in building a circle of people over time who shared that same faith is what guided my emotional stability. It helped me physically get well, too. I belonged to a great church during a lot of this. When I first got sick a lot of people at the new church did not know me. At first, we would go to church and then home. Around the time we got married and I had lost all of my hair, I went to a recovery group at church on a Monday night. I wore chemo caps because my scalp would burn a lot. The group was for all kinds of recovery, not just substance abuse or cancer. Well, I shared my story with them and started to meet people and I got 'prayer buddies.' They were people that I could count on to call on the phone and chit-chat and fill them in on what was going on with me. They were supportive and allowed me to put my faith in front of what was physically happening to me. I remember at the beginning of my illness being on my knees and just praying that God would help me. I'd be sobbing saying 'Please don't let me lose all my hair.' I had to learn to accept the situation. I mean I didn't feel that it was God's will that I would lose all my hair. I was not angry at my creator for that. I knew it was a problem with my immune system. I had to focus on being stable enough to let my body heal. I attribute my faith, the self-care that I did, and my mindset to focus on getting well as the things that helped me. I had to remind myself that we had to 'pump the brakes' and not overdo it for the sake of my health. We couldn't travel, and I also refrained from going out with my girlfriends because I knew that a late night could cause me to be on my butt for the next seven days wiped out. I told myself that for right now 'I just had to be' and that would have to be enough."

**Claudia** survived septic shock syndrome and the amputation of her leg. She recounted, "My family and my young adult children were there for me. I've always had a wonderful family and friends. They traveled to the local hospital where I was in the ICU and then traveled to Boston when I was transferred. They were by my side through the entire ordeal. I appreciate them even more now and I think they appreciate me even more. Everyone has been so attentive to me. People are always checking in on me. I never have to worry about anything. There are always people around to help. I am so blessed."

**Rose** survived a plane crash in Vietnam. She recounted, "My husband was the most supportive person, especially because we were newlyweds when I was in the plane crash. He was my rock in the months that followed. We grew even closer. He died a few years ago, but I can still recall how caring and supportive he was."

**Julie** was brutally mugged in New York City. She recalled, "My closest friends in NYC are my two girlfriends with whom I share an apartment. They are the best. They took care of me after I was released from the hospital. I can always count on them. It is very reassuring to have a supportive network of friends in NYC."

**Millicent** survived a serious postpartum hemorrhage. She related, "I have always had a very supportive network of family and friends. My women friends are awesome and strong. I also have a band of brothers and male friends. My husband, Larry, and I have a great marriage built on love and mutual respect. He is so supportive of me. We are fortunate to have found each other in this crazy world. He's my best friend and soul mate. He's a great husband and father. He's my one and only."

**Tara** was severely burned in a house fire. She remembered, "The reconstructive surgeries were approximately every six months up until I was around 18 years of age. My parents and my sister were so supportive. My sister homeschooled me for the first year after my injuries. My doctors, nurses, and therapists were so supportive, caring, and encouraging. These burn team members at the hospital were some of the greatest people I ever met in my entire life. They were professional but so loving, too."

**Sarah** survived three cardiac arrests in the ambulance on the way to the hospital. She described her homecoming when she was discharged from the hospital. Sara recalled, "When I walked into the house every relative was there to greet me. It was like a family reunion. I felt very loved and cared for. When I walked through the door, it was many emotions; some people were crying, and others cheering, and I felt so special. Some people were jumping up and down. They told me they couldn't believe what happened. I was lucky to be in an airport with a defibrillator. Friends and relatives were there for me. People brought meals over every day for the first month I was home. The generosity and caring were unbelievable. A lady from my church who cleaned houses cleaned my house every week and would not accept a dime for her services. I had an army of help, so I never felt alone."

## Theme: A Second Chance At Life

**Claudia** recovered from septic shock syndrome. She related, "I think I am a miracle because I got a second chance to live. The doctors said, 'We have never seen a blood infection so severe where anyone has survived.' I said, 'I know it was a miracle because a lot of people have been praying to God for me.' God spared my life for a reason. I think He realized that my children and grandchildren needed me. I think that I realized my strength, my faith, and my hope for the future. God is my Lord and Savior."

**Tara** had many surgeries to recover from being burned in a house fire. Tara reported, "God spared me. I have a great appreciation for life. I value life. I believe it is a gift. I survived for a reason. I treasure life and I move forward. I find that I have a strong belief in God. I am both religious and spiritual. I can rely on the grace of God. What occurs in my life and what has occurred in the past, I may not agree with or be happy about it, but God has always given me the grace to accept things and go on even if I don't understand the situation. I know that God will reveal things to me at a later time and then all of a sudden, I know why something happened. God points it out to me. I never questioned why I got burned. I never said, 'Why me?' There was an underlying acceptance. Of course, you don't want bad things to happen, but you don't question it. You can't control life events, and God has a plan for each of us."

**Cecilia** recalled, "I was spared a drowning death. I think that when you go through a traumatic event, you question what you are doing in your life. I questioned why I was spared. So many people die in the world, life is so fragile. After my almost drowning, I looked at the world differently. I was almost celebratory. In the months after the near-drowning, I saw things more clearly."

**Eve** was injured in a serious car crash. She related, "My relationships with family, friends, and co-workers have always been solid. However, after being injured in this horrible car accident, I was overwhelmed with the concern, caring, and kindness of others. I also don't sweat the small stuff anymore. I am so grateful for my second chance at life. My husband is an incredible man who has proved himself to me in so many ways. When we do have kids, I know that he'll be a wonderful father. I guess I have a great appreciation for those people who are close to me. I have always been a people person but even more so since the accident."

**Rose** survived a plane crash where many people were killed. Rose recalled, "I was saved while about half the people on the plane died. I survived and I believe in making the most of each day. I treasure my life and family and friends. I am grateful for surviving this horrible tragedy and for rejoining the Air Force after taking a few years off to process everything that happened."

**Julie** was mugged in New York City. She recounted, "I feel fortunate to have survived this brutal attack and been given another chance at living my life. After being a victim of a mugging, I have renewed compassion for all victims of crime. I also have compassion for those less fortunate: the homeless, the sick, the poor, the mentally ill, and others who find themselves in compromised circumstances. I hate to see innocent people hurt. I have become politically active to rally for increased law enforcement, crime victims' rights, and stricter gun control laws."

**Norma** was in critical condition, paralyzed, and on a ventilator from Guillain–Barre syndrome. She recalled, "My mind was unaffected, and I wondered if I would live or die. I came off the ventilator and could breathe on my own after about five weeks. I started to make significant progress, and I and my family began to think I would live and recover. I feel like my life is two chapters: before Guillain–Barre versus after Guillain–Barre. Now, I continue to live my 'second' life."

**Norma** continued, "I have had experiences of posttraumatic growth. I remember talking to our family attorney and his daughter was very sick in the hospital with Guillain–Barre syndrome. He said, 'Norma, I need you.' He talked to me on the phone from the hospital and said his daughter Maria was having trouble breathing. She was 25 years old. I took it upon myself to visit her every day for the next six months since I had battled Guillain–Barre syndrome and come out surviving on the other end. She finally had the ventilator removed, and I remember being so happy that I cried and cried and cried because it caused me to relive my own experience. She said, 'Thank you for helping me get through this experience.' Being with her helped her but it also helped me come to terms with my past. I was able to put things in perspective."

## Theme: I'm Stronger Than I Thought I Would Be

**Tara** was burned in a house fire at seven years of age. Tara stated, "I have personal strength. I believe that I am resilient. Part of it came from a time when I was younger and people said to me, 'You're never going to amount to anything in your life.' I could say to myself, 'I can be something in my life.' I knew that I was intelligent, smart, and capable. I've proved a lot of people wrong. I graduated with a 4.0 GPA from my bachelor's program, a 4.0 from my master's program, and a 4.0 from my doctorate program. I got the highest award from Hunter-Bellevue. I was reticent at first to go back for my bachelor's degree because I went to a diploma nursing school. I thought, 'Can I do this?' I answered, 'Yes I can!' I said to myself, 'You can do this.' I did not set myself up for failure. I moved ahead."

"Going back to school was certainly a new opportunity offering a new possibility. Eventually, a few people encouraged me to teach nursing. At first, I wasn't too sure about it. But I kept hearing this from different people. People thought I was a good teacher and good at explaining things to others. My Mom and Dad always believed in me. But I found out that others did, too. I had a passion and love for nursing. This also translated into a love for teaching student nurses. Others saw something in me that I didn't initially see in myself then."

**Millicent** survived a serious postpartum hemorrhage and needed six blood transfusions. She related, "I experienced posttraumatic growth as a result of living through this close brush with death. I recognized my strength as a woman, my high pain tolerance, my positive attitude, my faith in God, my belief in Mother Nature and the power of birth, and the importance of having a loving supportive partner to be with you in labor as well as in life. My midwives were there with me every step of the way, which is quite different from a doctor running in at the last minute to catch a baby. Midwives are guardians of the birth process. Midwife means 'with a woman.' Even when a woman experiences serious complications as I did, she can still feel good about her efforts and decisions. I am strong and I appreciate the life that God has given me."

**Eve** survived a serious car crash. She recalled, "My view of myself changed; in that, I realized that I was a strong person and a survivor. Before the accident, I had never been seriously ill or injured. I had a pretty happy and healthy life. Being incapacitated for a few months made me think about the past, the present, and the future. I wasn't used to resting so much and not being able to do things for myself. Besides my body healing, I think my mind healed and expanded as well. I started to think about how I wanted to spend the rest of my life. Of course, there were frustrations at times, and I could be impatient with my body at times. But I tried to focus on getting better and keeping a positive attitude. I think my spirituality grew as well, and I realized how someone's life can be snuffed away in a flash."

**Bambi** survived a serious cardiac infection. She reported, "I always felt as though I was a strong person, and this experience reinforced that. I feel even stronger now that I have recovered. I always felt strong and independent, and this experience helped me in my perception of self. Throughout my healing and recovery, I went on believing that I was a strong person and that I can take on things and make progress in reaching my physical, emotional, and career goals. Although there were peaks and valleys in the recovery process, and I was hospitalized for 57 days, I recovered and returned to work. I've had a very successful career as an educator."

### Theme: Putting the Pieces of My Life Back Together

**Julie** was mugged in New York City. She recalled, "It took me a long time to stop looking over my shoulder while walking home at night in NYC. However, this experience taught me a powerful lesson that you can never be too careful and that it is a lot easier to give up your purse than your life. I should not have hesitated to give him my purse because he could have had a knife or a gun. Maybe if I didn't struggle with him, he wouldn't have beaten me so much. It could have been worse; I could have been raped or killed. When something happens so fast, you don't have time to think. I am so grateful to be alive. I love my life in NYC. I have great friends there. I went to college in NYC and simply stayed there because I loved it. I do visit my family at Christmas and in the summer, but I consider NYC my home. I am a strong woman, and I didn't want the mugging to define me. Yes, I was an innocent victim that night, but I don't consider myself a perpetual victim. I have taken a self-defense class and have pepper spray. The kindness and caring of my two girlfriends were greatly appreciated. The three of us met in college and have been together since then. We look out for each other. We all try not to walk home alone, but sometimes it happens. We all carry pepper spray now. Sometimes we take taxi cabs, and we never take the subway at night."

**Samantha** survived a very long bout with Lyme disease. She related, "I always want to focus on my progress and not on negative things. When I would lose a handful of hair sometimes, my heart would be in my throat. You had to fight this desperate anxiety and say, 'I'm not going there again. I'm not doing this.' I would also sometimes have a massive fear of going hiking with my kids because of the risk of tick exposure. I had to rise above a lot of things and focus on progress and the positive things in my life. Also, when I was a new mom, I would be afraid of my kids getting a tick bite. But I learned to take precautions. We get our yard sprayed every six weeks from March to the end of September with pure cedar oil from a tick control company. I have slowly put my life back together, but it has been a prolonged venture over many years."

**Millicent**, who survived a serious postpartum hemorrhage, remarked, "This experience did not keep me from having other children. I simply put my faith in God that 'lightning would not strike twice.' I managed my fear and stress through prayer, meditation, and relaxation breathing. Although whenever I had a bleeding episode such as a heavy period or a nosebleed or a bad headache or felt faint, these occurrences reminded me of the postpartum hemorrhage. They served as triggers that brought me right back to the traumatic experience. They brought me back to my close brush with death. My husband was so worried about me. The whole experience of me bleeding profusely frightened him immensely. Years later, I read about EMDR therapy, which has helped some war veterans deal with trauma. Well, I tried it, and it did help me handle the triggers and stress responses to a certain extent. I would recommend it to others who have had PTSD, panic attacks, and intense traumatic experiences."

**Eve** was involved in a serious automobile accident. She recalled, "After I came home from the hospital, I had a lot of time to reflect on my life while I was recuperating from my injuries.

I started to think about what mattered to me, what was important in my life, and what I wanted to do in the future. I thought about the memories I had with family and friends, the holidays, vacations, and the fact that I loved my job. My life had been very good up until the accident. However, I was able to dig deeper into my thoughts while getting better. My husband was my 'rock,' and we had talked about starting a family in a year or so. I started to look for meaning in my life, and I wanted to continue on this path of discovery. I had so much time to think, and up until this point I had always been busy, busy, busy. So, having all this time to think and reflect was good for me. I was forced to slow down and not be my usual busy self. The accident and recovery period made me think more about the future in a very realistic way. This was good for me."

**Ivana** survived breast cancer and leukemia. She stated, "I've been in remission since 2015. I could go back, but I'm just hoping that I won't. I don't know if I would call it growth, but it altered my perspective on life. I remember before I got sick, Leo and I had thought about buying an apartment in NYC. Our plan was we'd live in NYC for the winters and stay up in the Hudson Valley during the summers. It would be milder, and we wouldn't have to deal with all the ice and snow. But after I recovered, I said, 'You know what, it is not worth it.' The thing that became the most important thing to me was family and friends. I said, 'I don't want to spend all this money to live in NYC and see shows and go to concerts; that's just not that important anymore. What I want is to see my family and friends and spend time with them.' I don't know whether you would call it growth, but it certainly is a change in perspective. It is a change in what is important now, and what is no longer important. Some people might call it growth."

**Norma** had a tough fight with Guillain–Barre syndrome and spent over a month paralyzed on a ventilator to breathe. She stated, "My view of myself changed after I recovered. Now, I love myself more. I have acquired 'a thick skin.' I am stronger than I thought I was. I know my limits and I have learned to say, 'No.' I have learned to ignore frivolous things. I know I can't fix everything. I have learned to prioritize things now. My son, Mitch, has had a big influence on me. He gave me a prayer book and I do the morning liturgy when I get up and I do the evening liturgy before I go to bed. I pray when I need something, and I also pray to thank God. I enjoy a very good and fulfilled life. I put God first, then, my family. I see myself as a voice for others who can't help themselves. I can see different perspectives. I am probably more conservative, too. I see myself as a patient advocate."

**Claudia**, who recovered from septic shock, meningitis, and lung and kidney failure, remarked, "They had put me on dialysis 24/7 for several days, and it worked. My lungs also came back. Now I have a few reminders. I had a below-the-knee amputation. The rehabilitation therapist thought I was too happy and too positive. They sent someone to talk to me because they thought I was in denial. I said, 'God spared my life, and I'll walk again even though I lost my leg.' The counselor said, 'You are not acting normal, you will have delayed grief.' I said, 'I'm not sad, I'm grateful.'"

### Theme: Near-Death Experiences... Some Women Had Them

**Sarah** had three cardiac arrests in the ambulance on the way to the hospital after collapsing in an airport. Sarah recalled, "After the event, I had dreams about it, and I must say that a very peaceful feeling comes over me. I was not feeling any pain but had a very complete feeling of peace. I think I knew I had a cardiac arrest. I had a fleeting memory, and it was something that I had never experienced before. It was such peace and calm. That's the only way I can describe it. I guess it was some type of near-death experience. I can't say that I saw a light or God but there was such calm and peace. I don't remember anyone doing anything to me or working on me, but I remember the motion of the ambulance. I wasn't scared, and I don't remember a vision; it was more of a feeling of calm and peace. It was amazing, and I can't put a name to it. I just remember the feeling of calm and peace."

**Bambi** was hospitalized in the Intensive Care Unit because of a cardiac infection that also involved her artificial pacemaker. Bambi remarked, "I was in the hospital for 57 days. One evening I was in bed and I visually saw what looked like a light chiffon scarf that waved in front of me. Then a nurse appeared. She saw something on one of the monitors. Then, all of a sudden, I heard the call for an RRT (rapid response team) to my room, and the room became flooded with people and lights. I remember hearing conversations, and the nurse in me knew some of the things they were saying and what they were doing. I remember hearing them say, 'Elevate her feet,' and I wanted to be a compliant patient, so I lifted my legs. Then, I continued to listen to the conversations as if I was hovering above myself and the professionals in the room. I kept thinking, 'What else can they do; start certain medications,' and then it was almost as if I went to sleep as a result of maybe some of the medications they were giving me. It was a peaceful sleep. I felt very calm. I was not panicked by the situation at all. Then, when I woke everyone was gone from the room. There was one nurse left, but there was no crowd. I felt okay. But it is an experience that I have thought about many times, and how fortunate I am to have the memory of it. The nurse in me recognizes the precarious situation I was in because there I was without a pacemaker monitoring me and really in danger to the point where they had to call this RRT to resolve the situation that had developed with my heart."

**Cecilia** almost drowned when she became entangled in her sweatshirt and went under. She was saved after her friends realized what was happening. She recalled, "I was at first panicked and fighting to get free of my tangled sweatshirt, then after a while, I felt peace. I felt a sense of relaxation. In front of me flashed different scenes of my life. And I know at 13 or 14 you don't have much of a sense of life. I saw my parents, I saw myself, I saw Thanksgiving, and I saw Christmas. These were all like flashes of my life through the years. I guess they were like things that were special to me. Then, all of a sudden, I don't remember anything after that. And, the next thing I know, I'm on the raft, the sweatshirt is off me, and people are working on me."

**Norma** was stricken with Guillain–Barre syndrome when she was in her 20s. Norma recalled, "I was on a ventilator for a month and unable to talk. Mentally I was with it. I remember one day the respiratory therapist forgot to turn on the ventilator alarm. The tubing filled with water, and the flow of oxygen stopped. I was completely out. I was in another place, and I was looking down from above, and all of a sudden, I heard people saying, 'Breathe, breathe, breathe,' and I came back. When I was gone, I was in this white place and I felt no pain, I felt completely loved and I was very happy. I don't know where I was, but I knew I was in a very special place. When they brought me back, I was angry. I went from feeling happy to feeling angry. Soon I became more talkative, especially when the vent was removed. I swear it took me 20 years to be able to put all of this together."

**TABLE 5.1** Women's Close Brush with Death Demographics

| Name | Age at Time of Close Brush with Death | Occupation | Type of Close Brush with Death |
|---|---|---|---|
| Claudia | 60 | Teacher | Septic shock, pneumonia, leg amputation, bacterial spinal meningitis, kidney failure, RSV |
| Tara | 7 | Professor | Severe burns in a house fire, 8 months in hospital, 26 reconstructive surgeries |
| Bambi | 63 | Nurse | 57 days in hospital/ICU for heart valve infection and infection on artificial pacemaker leads |
| Rose | 27 | Flight nurse | Plane crash where over 100 people were killed; sustained back and leg injuries |
| Julie | 28 | Theater usher | Mugged in New York City; sustained concussion, lacerations, and abrasions to face and neck |
| Sarah | 58 | Midwife | Had three cardiac arrests in the ambulance after collapsing at the airport |
| Millicent | 30 | Teacher | Had postpartum hemorrhage after delivering a healthy baby. Needed emergency D&C for retained placenta and six blood transfusions |
| Norma | 28 | Film producer | Paralyzed from Guillain–Barre syndrome. Spent over a month on a ventilator in ICU |
| Cecilia | 14 | Counselor | Near drowning experience in a lake |
| Samantha | 33 | Graduate student | Chronic Lyme disease, spontaneous pneumothorax, cardiac tamponade |
| Ivana | 66 | Biologist | Breast cancer. Developed acute leukemia from chemotherapy to treat breast cancer. Subdural hematoma from fall |
| Eve | 27 | Waitress | Car accident. Fractured leg, ankle, wrist, and facial lacerations |

The aforementioned testimonies reflect these women's strength, steadfast will to live, optimism, and determination in the face of adversity, and for some their abiding faith in God or a higher power. The support of their healthcare providers, family, co-workers, and friends, according to most of these traumatized women, played a significant role in their survival. Many were young when they faced medical emergencies such as near drowning, surviving a plane crash, or a mugging that put their lives in jeopardy. All of them cheated death but faced the physical and emotional challenges of surviving a close brush with death (see Table 5.1).

## References

Beck, C. T., & Watson, S. (2016). Posttraumatic growth after birth trauma. *MCN. The American Journal of Maternal/Child Nursing, 41*(5), 264–271. https://doi.org/10.1097/nmc.0000000000000259

Bryngeirsdottir, H. S., & Halldorsdottir, S. (2022). "I'm a winner, not a victim": The facilitating factors of post-traumatic growth among women who have suffered intimate partner violence. *International Journal of Environmental Research and Public Health, 19*(3), Article 1342. https://doi.org/10.3390/ijerph19031342

Greyson, B. (1983). The near-death experience scale: Construction, reliability, and validity. *Journal of Nervous and Mental Diseases, 171*(6), 369–375. https://doi.org/10.1097/00005053-198306000-00007

Khanna, S., & Greyson, B. (2015). Near-death experiences and posttraumatic growth. *Journal of Nervous and Mental Disease, 203*(10), 749–755. https://doi.org/10.1097/nmd.0000000000000362

Levy, K., Grant, P. C., Depner, R. M., Byrwa, D. J., Luczkiewicz, D. L., & Kerr, C. W. (2020). End-of-life dreams and visions and posttraumatic growth: A comparison study. *Journal of Palliative Medicine, 23*(3), 319–324. https://doi.org/10.1089/jpm.2019.0269

Martin, L., Byrnes, M., Bulsara, M. K., McGarry, S., Rea, S., & Wood, F. (2017). Quality of life and posttraumatic growth after adult burn: A prospective, longitudinal study. *Burns, 43*(7), 1400–1410. https://doi.org/10.1016/j.burns.2017.06.004

Martin, L., Byrnes, M., McGarry, S., Rea, S., & Wood, F. (2016). Evaluation of the posttraumatic growth inventory after severe burn injury in Western Australia: Clinical implications for use. *Disability and Rehabilitation, 38*(24), 2398–2405. https://doi.org/10.3109/09638288.2015.1129448

Martin, L. L., Campbell, W. K., & Henry, C. D. (2004). The roar of awakening: Mortality acknowledgment as a call to authentic living. In J. Greenberg, S. L. Koole, & T. Pyszsczynski (Eds.), *Handbook of experimental existential psychology* (pp. 431–448). Guilford Press.

Mehrabi, E., Hajian, S., Simbar, M., Houshyari, M., & Zayen, F. (2015). Posttraumatic growth: A qualitative analysis of experiences regarding positive psychological changes among Iranian women with breast cancer. *Electronic Physician, 7*(5), 1239–1246. https://doi.org/10.14661/1239

Oh, J. M., Kim, Y., & Kwak, Y. (2021). Factors influencing posttraumatic growth in ovarian cancer survivors. *Support Care Cancer, 29*(4), 2037–2045. https://doi.org/10.1007/s00520-020-05704-6

Peinkhofer, C., Dreier, J. P., & Kondziella, D. (2019). Semiology and mechanisms of near-death experiences. *Current Neurology and Neuroscience Reports, 19*(9), Article 62. https://doi.org/10.1007/s11910-019-0983-2

Royse, D., & Badger, K. (2017). Near-death experiences, posttraumatic growth, and life satisfaction among burn survivors. *Social Work in Health Care, 56*(3), 155–168. https://doi.org/10.1080/00981389.2016.1265627

Tedeschi, R., & Calhoun, L. (1995). *Trauma and transformation: Growth in the aftermath of suffering.* Sage.

Tedeschi, R. G., & Calhoun, L. G. (1996). The posttraumatic growth inventory: Measuring the positive legacy of trauma. *Journal of Traumatic Stress, 9*(3), 455–471. https://doi.org/10.1007/BF02103658

Tedeschi, R. G., & Calhoun, L. G. (2004). Posttraumatic growth: Conceptual foundations and empirical evidence. *Psychological Inquiry, 15*(1), 1–18. https://doi.org/10.1207/s15327965pli501_01

Wren-Lewis, J. (1994). Aftereffects of near-death experiences: A survival mechanism hypothesis. *Journal of Transpersonal Psychology, 26*, 107–115.

Zhai, J., Newton, J., & Copnell, B. (2019). Posttraumatic growth experiences and its contextual factors in women with breast cancer: An integrative review. *Health Care for Women International, 40*(5), 554–580. https://doi.org/10.1080/07399332.2019.1578360

# 6

# POSTTRAUMATIC GROWTH IN WOMEN WHO HAVE EXPERIENCED INTIMATE PARTNER ABUSE

Control is not love. Control is not protection or caring. Control is about power. It is about having another person under one's thumb or manipulating them in some way to do what the abuser commands. People can go through life tangled in a web of control and abuse which is dictated by their partner. The ebb and flow of abuse eats at one's basic core of dignity, self-respect, confidence, and motivation. In the United States it is estimated that one in three women are victims of abuse and that intimate partner violence is a leading cause of morbidity and mortality for women of childbearing age (Breiding et al., 2014). Survivors report long-term physical and psychological effects, including anxiety, depression, chronic illness, and debilitating lasting injuries (Black et al., 2011; Rivara et al., 2007).

This chapter describes the experience of intimate partner abuse encountered by women through the lens of the posttraumatic growth (PTG) model by Tedeschi and Calhoun (1996, 2004). It specifically addresses a gap in the abuse literature focusing on the development of PTG in women in the United States (Cobb et al., 2006).

## What Does the Research Tell Us?

Posttraumatic growth has been studied in various groups of trauma survivors. These groups include cancer survivors (Oh et al., 2021; Soo & Sherman, 2014), adult burn victims (Martin et al., 2017; Royse & Badger, 2018), amputees (Benetato, 2011), widows (Doherty & Scannell-Desch, 2021a), physically abused children (Farnia et al., 2017), traumatic childbirth survivors (Sawyer et al., 2012), combat soldiers and veterans (Larick & Graf, 2012; Mark et al., 2018; Palmer et al., 2016; Tsai et al., 2015), disaster survivors (Holgerson et al., 2010) and bereaved mothers (Doherty & Scannell-Desch, 2021b). There is an insufficient amount of research about PTG and abused women in the United States given the magnitude of the problem (Breiding et al., 2014).

Although intimate partner abuse can be inflicted by men or women, the focus of this chapter is on the abuse of women by their partners. Intimate partner abuse is a global problem that is well documented in the research literature. This violence can have serious consequences on a woman's physical and mental health, and in extreme cases it can

DOI: 10.4324/9781003456650-6

result in a woman's death. Over the last 20 years, a small body of mostly qualitative research has emerged about abuse experiences and women's capacity for healing (Cobb et al., 2006; Gerber et al., 2012; Moschella et al., 2018).

In a mixed-method study, Anderson and colleagues (2012) explored the outcomes and recovery process of 37 women in an abusive relationship. Analysis revealed how social and spiritual support was essential in women's recovery and development of PTG. These findings are consistent with the current study, in that social support and faith-based activities brought the women comfort and aided in their healing.

Although only a few published US studies have explored PTG in abused women, some European and Asian researchers have studied PTG in women survivors of intimate partner abuse. In a quantitative French study, Magne and associates (2021) evaluated PTG in 17 women survivors of partner abuse and 42 women survivors of other types of violence. Participants were administered the 21-item Posttraumatic Growth Inventory (PTGI) (Tedeschi & Calhoun, 1996) and the 20-item Posttraumatic Stress Checklist (PCL-5) (Blevins et al., 2015). Findings indicated a higher percentage of PTG in survivors of partner abuse (82%) when compared with survivors of sexual assault (52%) and other types of interpersonal violence (53%). All five domains of PTG resulted in higher scores on the PTGI (Tedeschi & Calhoun, 1996) in women survivors of partner abuse when compared to the other two groups. This finding demonstrated the ability of the abused women group to withstand their adversity, trauma, and stress while developing PTG. These investigators found a clear negative correlation between PTG and PTSD (Magne et al., 2021).

In a study of 217 Filipino women who had reported partner abuse, Arandia and colleagues (2016) assessed the one-factor, three-factor, and five-factor PTG models to ascertain which model best described their sample. Findings demonstrated that the five-factor model (Tedeschi & Calhoun, 2004), which included appreciation of life, personal strength, spiritual change, new possibilities, and relating to others, best fit their sample. Moreover, every domain of the five-factor model was found to be positively correlated with the cognitive processing of trauma. Findings acknowledged the robustness and flexibility of the five-factor PTG model (Arandia et al., 2016).

Gonzalez-Mendez and Hamby (2020) examined the strengths associated with well-being and PTG in 109 Spanish women who had experienced intimate partner abuse. Participants completed a survey measuring multiple categories of strengths, personal well-being, and PTG. Two patterns were identified. One pattern showed some strength across the domains of PTG, and the other pattern showcased the women with high PTG scores. The results of this study suggested ways to enhance the well-being of these abuse survivors (Gonzalez-Mendez & Hamby, 2020). Findings revealed that PTG was positively correlated with well-being and all strengths listed on their survey instrument. While it is of utmost importance to promote safety for women, the current study explored the various facets of what helps some women to move their lives forward in a positive direction once the abuser is out of the household.

In a Polish study, Dyjakon and Rajba (2021) examined the experience of abuse and PTG changes in 48 women who reported partner abuse and were undergoing partner therapy. Inclusion criteria were having stayed in a relationship with a partner who used violence and the requirement that the partner also begins therapy aimed at changing the violent behavior. These investigators used the Impact Event Scale-Revised (IES-R) (Weiss & Marmar, 1996) and the PTGI (Tedeschi & Calhoun, 1996) to assess PTG. Findings demonstrated that over 18 months significant changes in PTG occurred. Results indicated that participants and their partners had undertaken therapy and made positive changes in their lives and that building a close relationship with the individual who caused the abuse can change the level of PTG. Changes in self-perception and changes in relating to others decreased over time, while an appreciation of life increased over time and spiritual life remained the same. According to the women, the violence had stopped, and their sense of security had increased significantly (Dyjakon & Rajba, 2021). The current study did not address partner therapy because only one of 14 women remained in a relationship with her partner.

## Our Study Themes

Five themes were formulated from narrative interview data from women who have experienced intimate partner abuse: (1) acknowledging the abusive relationship; (2) fear of him: threats, control, pain, and isolation; (3) accepting support: grabbing the life preserver; (4) rediscovering myself: digging deep; and (5) appreciating life and helping others.

## Our Study Methods

Similar to our previously cited studies in this book exploring the experiences of widows, women who have lost a child, and women who have had a close brush with death, this study about intimate partner abuse employed purposive and snowball sampling to recruit women who met the study inclusion criteria. Inclusion criteria consisted of women who reported emotional and/or physical abuse to a nursing provider; the ability to read, write, and speak English; the ability to recall experiences of abuse; and willingness to discuss their abuse experiences. Participants were recruited through the investigators' nursing network, which consisted of faculty and clinical colleagues. Institutional Review Board approval was granted by the university where the first author was employed.

Potential participants who met the inclusion criteria were mailed a letter explaining the study and the concept of PTG. A consent form and return mailing envelope were included for those interested in participating in the study. Fourteen consent forms and demographic information sheets were completed and returned. After written consent was obtained, an email was sent to schedule an interview at the participant's convenience. Data were collected from the Fall of 2020 through the Fall of 2021. A mental health nurse practitioner was available for debriefing if any participant became upset or felt uncomfortable during or after the interview. None of the participants needed debriefing, counseling, or a referral for further services. Many said it was cathartic and helpful to share their story of abuse with nurse researchers. All interviews were audio-recorded for accuracy and transcribed verbatim.

When interviewing clients who experienced intimate partner abuse, the client's safety needs to be of paramount importance as well as her privacy. Assessment and discussion of intimate partner abuse need to be in a private setting, whether it is an in-person assessment or a virtual one using telehealth or another technological method (Doyle et al., 2022). In the current study, only one woman was still living with her husband. We ensured that she chose a date and time for her speaker-phone interview when her husband was out of town.

The overarching research question was: What are women's experiences of partner abuse, and did they experience posttraumatic growth over time? Participants were asked the following interview questions: (1) Describe your experience of abuse in detail. (2) Describe any experiences you would consider to be PTG. (3) Describe any changes in your relationships with family and friends. (4) Describe any sense of compassion or empathy for others. (5) Describe any changes you see in yourself. (6) Describe your current philosophy of life. (7) Is there anything else you would like to tell me? The researchers took field notes to document emotional reactions such as crying or sighing.

Narrative data were analyzed by qualitative content analysis (Cleland, 2017; Sandelowski, 2009). Audio recordings were listened to several times to gain familiarity with the tone and content. Significant phrases and statements were extracted and sorted to form theme clusters. Both researchers reviewed and coded each transcript separately to gain rigor (Cleland, 2017; Hays & Singh, 2011). Then, they worked collaboratively to achieve consensus on thematic data placement. In a qualitative study, researchers are particularly concerned with the trustworthiness of the data. Rigor was strengthened by attending to credibility, confirmability, dependability, and transferability (Hays & Singh, 2011). Credibility and confirmability were enhanced by audio recording and verbatim transcriptions (Lincoln & Guba, 1985). Thick descriptions, which are considered rich and detailed descriptions, were abundant in the narrative data and were integrated into the findings to strengthen transferability. An audit trail, field notes, and a thematic decision list helped to ensure the dependability of findings.

The 14 participants ranged in age from 40 to 80, and the mean age was 57.7 years at the time of the interview. Years of abuse varied from 6 years to 60 years (in the case of the one woman who was still married). Two women had no children, others had between one and three children, and the woman who was still married had eight children. One woman had adopted two children after her divorce. All women reported being in the middle socioeconomic class and had at least a high school diploma, and many had an associate or baccalaureate degree. Each participant was assigned a pseudonym for confidentiality.

### Theme: Acknowledging the Abusive Relationship

Women reported how they came to terms with recognizing that they were in an abusive relationship. They described an element of sadness and defeat even if they wanted out of the relationship. They related that it was difficult to give up on something that had been wanted and valued earlier. When children were involved, women realized that ties might not be completely severed. A cleaner break could usually be made if there were no children or if the children were adults. The realization of abuse did not come without pain and heartbreak. The following excerpts from the women's stories support this theme.

#### Sabrina and Antonio

**Sabrina** stated, "I was with my boyfriend at the time, who is my daughter's father. I met Antonio during my freshman year of college at the age of 18, and I was with him till 25 years of age when I left. Through those years I experienced mental and physical abuse. It started even before I had my daughter with little things like arguing or him grabbing me. He always wanted to be in control of everything, which included me. He was an only child but raised predominantly by his grandmother, who had 17 children. He was the baby, and they spoiled him rotten. He was a big basketball player for Virginia. That's where I went to college. He was always used to getting his way, and his mom would have him visit for Christmas and holidays, and she was working hard. So, his grandmother raised him. I can't understand why he was the way he was. There could have been abuse in the family, I didn't know. It escalated to slapping me or just not being around for days. When I had the baby, I couldn't depend on him if at times he just wasn't around. I continued to go to school, and I stayed down there even though my whole family was in New York. When he came around it was almost more harm than good. It was almost like me taking care of him and the baby. If he didn't like what I cooked, he would get mad. I remember one time he took a whole pan of bacon and threw it down the hill. I was barely surviving, and he takes the whole pan of bacon and throws it down the hill."

**Sabrina** continued, "He was a womanizer, too. I went to California with him because that's where his mother lived. I also don't know why I continued to stay in this relationship. I remember lots of times when he would be abusive. I remember one time he came home and I guess I didn't act happy to see him and he just ripped the nightgown right off me and then shredded the book I was reading. I was so distraught because it was my boss's book. Here I was working, taking care of my daughter, and trying to keep everything together. He would snicker at me, criticize me, mock me. It was like I was never good enough. I did leave him when our daughter was four. It was almost like a movie; I planned my escape. I knew he was going out, and I got all my things and my daughter's things together. I knew he was out cheating, and I knew I was getting a decent paycheck. My boss helped me. We put all my stuff and my daughter's stuff in these big garbage bags. I slept at my boss's house because the train I was going to take across the country to the east coast from California was on a Saturday, so I stayed over on a Friday when I knew he'd be out. I also knew if he caught me doing this, I was probably going to lose my life."

"He caught me on the train. His mother told him where I was going to be. I love his mother dearly, but it surprised me that she would do this. He was just begging me not to leave. He cried and begged. He said, 'Don't do this to our family.' But I left. I went home for four months, but I did come back. It took us four and a half days on the train. Everybody loved my daughter on the train. She's a good kid. When I first went to California, it was the two of us driving cross country. She was used to traveling with me. She could adapt to anything. To this day, I don't know why I went back to California. He promised me he'd go to counseling, and somehow, I just wanted it to work with my daughter's father. I think everyone expected it not to work, and I wanted it to work. He said you left on a train so come back on a train. I don't know why he just didn't pay for us to fly. It would have been easier. The second I saw him, I knew deep, deep in my soul that I had made a mistake. During the three months I was back there he was 'good.' He didn't sleep around and didn't put his hands on me, but I couldn't stand him. I was indifferent to him. He was still doing whatever he wanted even if he didn't sleep around. I had made a decision. I planned a trip home, and I think he knew this time that I wasn't coming back. So, two weeks before I was going to return to New York, he was working as a security guard at a church and asked me to bring him some food. When I arrived, he grabbed the car keys from me. If I had to, I would have walked five miles to get out of there. He socked me so hard in my face that I fell to the ground. I was alone in the building with him. He was the security guard. I thought he was going to finish me off, but he got paged for his job, which probably saved my life. He had to answer the page, so I took the keys and ran to my car and drove to my apartment. I grabbed my hamper and knew that I had clothes in the hamper. He left work and came and blocked me in. My neighbor saw us and sensed something was going on, and she would not leave me. She knew something was up, so he finally left. I drove to his mother's house, and she was crying because she knew that he was giving me a hard time. So, I stayed at his mother's house for the last two weeks. He took the car, he took the keys, he took everything. I waited at my apartment for the mail because I was expecting a paycheck. Then I went back to his mother's. She kicked him out of the house. His mother bought Easter outfits for me and my daughter, and we went to church. She said, 'He's not going to keep you down.' She gave us a ride to the airport the day we were leaving. I did not shed a tear because I knew I was doing the right thing. I did not want my daughter to learn that men can treat women this way. I had shielded her from a lot of his bad behavior. That is probably what gave me the inner strength to do all of this and leave. I guess I wanted a better life for my daughter."

**Sabrina** continued, "I remember little things. That man was so abusive. He came to my job once because we were having an argument and he was harassing me, and I threw the phone at him. He was a calculating guy and waited four to five days and came to my job as if he was taking me out to lunch and hit me, pulled my hair, and said 'That's for throwing the phone.' I was so shaken up and crying and then had to go back to work in that condition. Over the years, he has hurt me more than my daughter. He didn't send child support and did all kinds of mean and cruel things. I could cry right now because I am still so ashamed of this chapter of my life. I am so ashamed that I allowed a person to treat me that way."

### Joanne and Theo

**Joanne** recalled, "Theo's controlling behavior started gradually after we were married. He was a successful lawyer with a big ego, and at first, I thought he was being a protective husband, which was admirable. However, this behavior escalated over the years into strict control over me and our daughter. Sometimes he engaged in 'gaslighting,' which made me doubt myself. By this I mean he would try to make me feel forgetful, confused, and like I was going crazy. This was subtle at first but grew over time. I would second guess myself a lot, feel uncertain about things, and insecure. Yet, before I married Theo, I was a world traveler as a seasoned flight attendant. I loved my job and grew to be senior with Pan American Airlines. I was responsible, fun-loving, and maybe slightly carefree. Life was an adventure for me, and I loved art galleries, theater, fashion, and cooking, and was a real people person. Yet, marriage and motherhood were my goals, and I was ready to settle down and put down some roots. I loved staying home and raising June. I met other moms and had a nice social circle. We arranged play dates for the kids and enjoyed coffee together and sometimes lunch. I was fortunate that Theo made enough money so that I could stay home and raise our daughter. June meant the world to us because I had secondary infertility after having her and never became pregnant again."

**Joanne** continued, "Theo was always orderly, organized, and meticulous in his work, in the way he dressed, and in the way he wanted our home to be. Let's face it, with kids, messes happen. He also considered himself an 'expert on parenting.' You couldn't tell him anything. He had an answer for everything. It didn't matter that I was with June all day and knew her habits, likes, and dislikes. Theo thought he was a younger version of Dr. Spock. This was ironic because he had one sister and a few cousins, and had never babysat or even been a camp counselor. How could someone consider themselves an expert when they had no experience in this domain? To his credit, he did read books on parenting and did want to be a good father. Things in our home were dictated by Theo's moods, ideas, legal work, and social obligations. I made no demands on him other than being a husband and father. Yet, he ruled with an 'iron hand,' meaning that decisions tended to be 'his way or the highway.' He always wanted to know where I was and what I was doing. He wanted to make sure I was making all of June's baby food and whom we were meeting with as 'Moms & Tots.' He wanted to 'approve' the books I read to June, the toys she played with, and the kids she was with. It was control, control, control. Control like this was not love or concern or caring; it was a form of abuse. Over the years, I felt like I was in prison or that I was the child and Theo was the parent. I think I put up with this for so many years for June's sake. I wanted her to grow up with a mother and a father."

**Joanne** added, "I always felt like I was under Theo's thumb so to speak. I lost myself in the process. I was no longer the capable woman Theo married. Life was so much better when I was with June and other mothers and kids. I started to dread going home because Theo interrogated me, criticized me, and put me down with his harsh comments. I had no real voice at home, yet I was still able to have enjoyable times with June and other moms and kids. Then when Theo had a bad day in court, he would yell and curse and blame everyone else related to the case. I would take June into her bedroom, and we would stay there for hours reading and playing. Theo's outbursts frightened me at times, and I didn't want June to become fearful of her Dad. Occasionally during one of his outbursts, he'd throw something at me. Fortunately, I was good at ducking or moving out of the way. I'd let him have his temper tantrum alone, and I'd whisk June away with me."

"Eventually, Theo started a solo law practice and had an office in our town rather than commuting to Chicago. Part of me thinks his decision was because he started having difficulty getting along with the other lawyers and paralegals in his firm. He never admitted that but said he was tired of having to listen to other people and preferred his own company. Theo thought he was an authority on everything, and I think this ruined some relationships along the way with friends, neighbors, relatives, and legal colleagues."

"I think I finally realized when June was older that I had no life of my own in terms of making decisions for myself without 'getting permission' from Theo. He refused to go to marriage counseling, saying that they couldn't tell him anything he didn't already know."

**Joanne** shared, "When June finally went away to college, it was my time to exit. I filed for divorce, and Theo exploded in a fit of anger. He cursed, called me horrible names, and threw things, breaking vases and glassware. He said that he gave me a 'charmed life' because I didn't have to work, lived in an affluent town, and had a nice house with a swimming pool and deck. I told him that I was a prisoner in my own home and that my self-esteem was in the toilet. I told him that I put up with his controlling behavior for too long, that I had lost myself in the process, and that I only stayed in the marriage to provide stability for June. On my own, I got a job as a travel agent and French teacher. June has accepted the situation and maintains a good relationship with both of us. She is much closer to me, though."

### Marcella and Wyatt

**Marcella** reported, "One day when my husband was away on a business trip, I was watching a detective show on the TV, and it dealt with marital abuse. It finally dawned on me that Wyatt's angry and hurtful words, lies, cruelty, and occasional pushing and shoving were abuse. I realized that I was living in an abusive relationship, and this was not normal."

**Marcella** continued, "I married my college sweetheart. I loved him with all my heart. He was an officer in the Navy. The first inkling that I had about his controlling behavior was the day after our wedding as we drove to Virginia. He gave me orders to be in the car at 7:30 AM. It was the day after our wedding, and I had hoped to sleep in, make love, cuddle, and start our married life on a romantic note. I was a virgin until our wedding night, a good Catholic girl who consciously saved herself for marriage even though I certainly had my share of boyfriends in high school and college. I remember thinking, 'How could he be so inconsiderate and demanding?' He was on shore leave for more than a week, so there was no rush to get to Virginia. Yet he was adamant about his request. I remember thinking to myself, 'Was my Doctor Jekyll turning into Mr. Hyde?' I fought tears as we drove all day to reach Virginia; this was my marriage introduction."

**Marcella** continued, "I was married to Wyatt for five years, and I truly loved him. However, he could be a very difficult and complicated person. His moods could change in a flash. He could be nice, thoughtful, charming, and fun one minute and then turn into an angry, brooding man the next minute. This tended to happen when things in life were not going his way. He was an extreme narcissist, very self-centered, cold, distant, arrogant, and lacking empathy for others. These behaviors were so opposite to my loving and caring nature as a special education teacher. However, when Wyatt had a problem and wanted to tell me about it, I always listened, supported him, and tried to help him."

**Marcella** added, "I distinctly remember Wyatt telling me that he did not know if he could ever love me as much as I loved him. He said this after we were married less than two weeks. It was a random comment as I was standing on a chair in the kitchen getting food items down from a high cabinet. I almost fell off the chair with his remark. He countered his remark by saying that the Navy came first, and I came second. I was in tears and extremely hurt by his comment. We were having friends over for dinner that night, and I remember trying to collect myself and put on a happy face."

"Surprisingly, Wyatt left the Navy after five years to go to graduate school. He had been stationed on a ship in Japan for a year, so I was not allowed to go with him. The Navy had its rules. I used the time to get a graduate degree. While he was in Japan, he became involved with a Japanese woman. There may have been more women, too. I did not know this information at the time; it was revealed to me much later. While abroad, I thought Wyatt was true to me, and I received love letters almost every day. He also sent me gifts and flowers. I honestly did not suspect infidelity."

**Marcella** reported, "We moved to New York City for graduate school. I found a good teaching job while he was in school. I thought this might be a new beginning for us, but it wasn't. Although he did well in graduate school, he was very moody and stressed most of the time. I did everything he asked me to do such as edit his papers, host his study group at our apartment, and attend social functions with him. Yet sometimes he made me feel like a servant, a Barbie doll, and a trophy wife. Everything was about him and his needs. I felt invisible and hurt. It was as if my purpose in life was to cater to his whims. Because I loved him, I put up with this treatment. I rationalized it in my mind and made excuses for his bad behavior. I knew he was stressed, tired, and possibly depressed. I tried to fulfill all his needs such as sex, maintaining a social presence, bringing in a salary, cooking, and cleaning. All I expected was to be treated decently and with respect. Wyatt could have a temper when things did not go his way, and he took it out on me. I didn't have black eyes or bruises, but there were times when he yelled at me and backed me up to the wall or shoved me when he was trying to make a point. A few times he grabbed my arm as I tried to get away from him. I grew to be afraid of him and his moods. I was afraid that he'd fly off the handle and push me off the balcony. I noticed that my body would tense up as I drove home from work each day as I got closer to our apartment building. I never knew what I was going to walk into: Would he treat me okay, or would he be in one of his dark moods? Sometimes he didn't even talk to me or acknowledge that I came home from work."

"One night in January of his second semester we were in bed, and he announced to me that there was something wrong with him. He told me that he had made an appointment with the school's psychiatrist. He said, "I don't know what's the matter with me because I have the most wonderful wife in the world but I don't want to have a wife anymore." He added, "You want kids, and I don't but I know I promised you that we would have them." I was crushed, devastated, and heartbroken to say the least. This announcement came out of the blue and hit me like a ton of bricks. My body shook as I sobbed in his arms, and he held me tight realizing that he had shattered my world. To make a long story short, the school psychiatrist sent him for intensive therapy with another psychiatrist who could see him three times a week. I prayed that Wyatt would get the help he needed. He was diagnosed with a narcissistic personality and a character disorder. Supposedly, he lacked compassion and empathy and didn't know how to love others."

**Marcella** shared, "After months of intensive therapy, I met with his psychiatrist, and he told me to let Wyatt go and 'run for the hills.' Wyatt wanted a no-fault divorce. He served me with papers at work. I divorced him on the grounds of cruel and abusive treatment and adultery. He didn't contest it. I then sought an annulment of our marriage in the Catholic church. Wyatt was not Catholic. Wyatt had confessed to a close male friend all of his indiscretions over dinner at a restaurant in NYC when the friend tried to talk some sense into him when we were heading toward a divorce. This man was a close friend of ours, and he served as a witness in the annulment proceedings. Not only was Wyatt lying and cheating during our marriage, but he had a few flings while we were engaged and he was away with the Navy. I was devastated to find out the truth because I would never have married him if I knew he was a cheater. He betrayed me. He was a con man, a phony."

**Marcella** concluded, "I remember asking Wyatt before we divorced about all the love letters he wrote to me while he was in Japan, and he replied, "It was a writing exercise." I think that says it all about this man's lack of integrity and inability to care about another human being. He was not capable of true love, so I had no choice but to walk away. Although I was heartbroken and had PTSD for years, I learned from this experience. I married Wyatt for the right reasons and truly wanted to build a family with the man I thought I knew from college. However, I was deceived, and his true colors came out as soon as I said, 'I do.' I became his possession, not his wife. Control, stonewalling, and gaslighting behaviors were paramount in Wyatt's modicum of behavior toward me. As painful as it was, I am so glad I escaped his narcissistic clutches. There is a part of me that feels sorry for him because he will probably never know true love. He does not have a conscience. Who can trust a person like that?"

### Bethany and Jordan

**Bethany** recalled, "I met my husband in graduate school. I think three men in my class were interested in me. I quickly dismissed the one who was married, but the two single guys both seemed nice. However, Jordan pursued me and won me over. When I met

Jordan, I had been divorced for two years. I did not date at all during those two years because I wanted to get over my bitterness. I had worked hard to get my self-esteem back. I had felt sad about not being in a loving relationship and prayed a lot for healing, which helped. Jordan certainly let me know that 'he picked me.' I felt strong and healed. He said that he knew 'I was the one,' and he had previously lived with three different women looking for the right one and I was 'the right one.' He accepted that I had a young son and said that he wanted to have children, too."

"Professionally, I was at the top of my game and I stayed there. Getting my doctorate was the next logical step for me. I was renting an apartment with my young son near Philadelphia. Jordan was five years older than me; he was 40 and I was 35. I remember being at a grad school gathering where he hovered over me, which was very flattering at the time. When we went back to my apartment, he never really left. He was living in a dorm room at the time. He had just had a kidney stone removed and asked if he could recuperate at my apartment. I said 'Yes.' So, here I am cooking for him, taking care of him, cleaning the apartment, working, and going to school.

We confided in each other, and I told Jordan about being treated poorly by my first husband. Jordan behaved just the opposite. He was loving, kind, and considerate. He told me that he had been abused by a camp counselor as a child."

**Bethany** continued, "To make a long story short, Jordan manipulated me right from the start. I came to realize over time that he had lied to me about many things. When he told me that he had lived with three different women, in truth, it was more like nine different women. He lied continuously, and I basically 'went from the frying pan into the fire.' There were signs which I now refer to as 'minefields.' He told me that he grew up in NYC and was a licensed counselor and psychologist. He told me that he had written a book, which I later found out was a blatant lie. He also told me that he had lived and studied in Paris but left without getting his Ph.D. He left to pursue a counseling opportunity in the Alaskan bush, which I thought was very humanitarian. What I found out much later was that he lived with a 15-year-old female drug addict in Alaska. This information was revealed to me when she demanded child support for the child they had together."

**Bethany** added, "Looking back on our 13-year marriage, I feel like I was such a fool to believe his lies. I remember soon after we met, he demanded 'exclusive dating.' I thought that was a sign that he loved me and didn't want to be with anyone else. He wanted me to meet his family, and we went to a post-Christmas party in NYC with about 15 people. There, in front of all these people, he asked me to marry him. He put this fake diamond on my ring finger. I was shocked, embarrassed, and horrified that he put me on the spot like this. I didn't know what to do so I said, 'Yes.'"

"We got married the following November. I did see some 'red flags,' and my mother tried to convince me and talk me out of it. Before we got married, I almost broke up with him several times. He had this high opinion of himself as an intellectual. We went together on a class trip to Cuba, and I started to see the worst in him. When I'd confront him on his behavior, he'd tell me, 'I'm working on it.' He also told me that his urologist who cared for him with the kidney stone had told him that it would be hard for him to father children, so he convinced me to try to get pregnant right away. I remember him saying, 'Let's try now.' Well, this turned out to be outright deception because I got pregnant instantly. I had two kids with him, Charles and Carla.

Jordan was manic-depressive; he was severely bipolar. He was an impossible man to live with, and I behaved like a fucking Mother Teresa taking care of him. In his eyes, I never gave him enough. He was also mean at times to my five-year-old son by my first marriage. He was okay with Charles and Carla."

**Bethany** reported, "Finally, I found out that he had been in therapy for a good part of his life but lied about it. His erratic behaviors were confusing, and he was diagnosed with a narcissistic personality disorder. He never made any progress in therapy because he lied about everything. He lied to his therapist. How can anyone make progress in therapy if they are not honest with their therapist?"

"He torpedoed my self-esteem and said things like, 'You are divorced with a kid. No one else will want you.' He convinced me and shamed me. He was controlling and jealous of my family and friends. I remember him telling me that 'no one can call you when I'm at home.' He was trying to cut me off from other people. He wanted me to feel sorry for him and said that his father had sexually abused his sister. He told me that he told his therapist that I was cold and withdrawn. He told things to his therapist over a 10-year period that were simply not true. He put me down at every chance he could get."

"I recall Jordan trying to get our son, Charles, to go on a fishing trip with him. Jordan wanted it to be a 'bonding experience.' Charles said, 'I hate Daddy and don't want to go on a fishing trip with him, I hate him.' This was probably the result of Jordan being loud at times and exhibiting odd behaviors. The kids got mixed messages. They saw him verbally abuse me many times. He was always mad at me. Yet, he would say, 'I love you and I love the kids.'"

"Jordan would go to Europe to teach. He would invite himself to different institutes and universities, but he would pay for it himself. I guess I was paying for it, too. For a long time, I wanted to leave Jordan. He would even say that he would go to an institution for treatment if I stayed with him."

**Bethany** shared, "When things got really bad, he would try to win me back. I tried and I would give, give, and give and never take. He had nothing to give me back. Staying with him was more harmful than good for me and the kids. The reason I stayed as long as I did was Irish Catholic guilt. We got divorced when the kids were seven and nine years old. I remember my kids saying that if we got divorced, they wanted to stay with me."

### Andrea and Mike

**Andrea** recalled, "I always knew that Mike liked to get together with friends and have a few beers after work or on weekends, but I didn't know this habit or addiction would escalate over time. It eventually made life difficult for me and our three kids. To a certain extent, I think I was in denial, and I think when the kids reached the age of ten, they were also in denial. My kids told me that other neighborhood kids would say mean things to them when they saw the truck from the brewery in our driveway. This occurred about once a week."

**Andrea** stated, "I am a social worker, so I knew about alcoholism. I knew that social drinking could lead to alcoholism if it increases. In retrospect, I think Mike was what you call a 'functioning alcoholic' because he never missed a day of work as a carpenter. Also, he only drank beer. I don't even remember him having a hangover. However, after a six-pack of beer, he could sometimes get annoyed or nasty. If the kids were noisy or not doing as he told them to quiet down or do their homework, off would come his leather belt. He would often say, 'You snot-nosed kids, you are never going to amount to anything.' If I got in the way of the belt, I got it too. I don't think Mike meant to hit me intentionally, but if I was in the line of fire, I got hit too. I remember my daughter, Maria, going to high school with a fat lip because the metal fastener of the belt got her in the lip. It was not that she did anything wrong, Mike was just in a bad mood and the kids were making noise, which set him off."

"I think the kids were relieved to go off to college and be away from their dad's drinking and temper. Yet all three kids loved their dad immensely when he was not drinking. He could be fun and was heavy into sports, especially baseball. He was also excellent at his craft, had a great singing voice, and played the piano. He was a very kind and generous person who helped others, too. He just wasn't his normal self when he was drinking. He could be very nasty and mean-spirited. We were afraid because he was not his normal self."

"As a social worker, I should have been more assertive in getting Mike some help, but I knew he'd refuse because he didn't think drinking beer was a big deal. Yet, it changed his personality, his demeanor, and his patience with others. Fortunately, he did not drink and drive. I didn't want to 'rock the boat' at home with more arguing or him getting annoyed with the kids and reverting to hitting them with a belt. So, often I kept quiet, made excuses for him, and covered up his bad behavior. I am a peacemaker, and I wanted my kids to be happy and have a normal home life. I swept a lot of unpleasantness under the rug so to speak. The web of denial was my protective mechanism. I guess I enabled Mike to be a mean alcoholic in some ways, but I just felt paralyzed trying to raise three kids with an alcoholic husband. The saga ended when Mike died of a heart attack in the hospital. We were all heartbroken and sad, but there was also an element of relief."

### Rosemary and Anthony

**Rosemary** stated, "After being married for over 50 years and having eight children together, you would think he'd treat me better than he does. He doesn't beat me up or anything like that, but he treats me poorly at times. He's mean, inconsiderate, and controlling and puts me down when he's angry or frustrated about things. He calls me names and gives me 'the silent treatment.' Once, I think he didn't talk to me for a month. And he does this thing called 'gaslighting.' There was a movie made about it many years ago where the husband was trying to drive the wife crazy. It's like this game he plays making me think I'm forgetting things or imagining things. He makes me question myself about what I am thinking or remembering or doing. Sometimes it makes me confused, and I start to doubt myself. The women in my church group talked about that movie. We talk about things in life because our husbands are not there. We are all senior citizens, and we share stories and compare notes sometimes. It's a close-knit group, and we've all known each other for years."

"I don't recall the exact year that I started to notice Anthony's bad behavior toward me. It was probably after we already had three or four kids, and we have eight in total. I guess eight kids in 18 years is a lot. Money was tight, and I was a stay-at-home Mom. I guess Anthony felt like the entire financial burden was on him. However, I could stretch a dollar as no one could. Also, my older sister was very good to me, and she didn't have any children. She'd help out occasionally, and I could always go to her if I needed a little extra money, and I would never tell Anthony because I knew he would resent it and get mad. My younger brother would sometimes take the kids places on Saturdays or Sundays because we lived in NYC. He would take them out for hamburgers or pizza or ice cream. They'd also go to Central Park or Bryant Park or Times Square back in those days. Sometimes he'd take them bowling or to a movie."

**Rosemary** continued, "When Anthony would get angry, he'd take off his belt and hit the kids. I would get hit if I got in the way of trying to protect the kids. No one got beaten up, just a thrash with the belt here and there. The kids were pretty good running in different directions when their Dad was on one of his rampages to escape getting hit with the belt. At times like this, none of us could do anything right in Anthony's eyes. I think his anger came from a tough upbringing. He didn't grow up in a kind household where people demonstrated their love for each other. His parents were rather cold and lacked good communication, but they did provide the basics for their kids: food, shelter, and clothing."

"As a husband and father of eight, I think Anthony often felt the weight of the world on his shoulders as he worked to support ten of us. Often, he took the joy out of our family life. The kids didn't like it when we argued or when 'the silent treatment' was happening. I don't mean to imply that our family life was horrible, but it just could have been a lot better. Anthony was the unpleasant person in the house, and he set the tempo for the rest of us. He was the breadwinner, and he never let anyone forget it."

"Even as we grew older as a married couple and the kids were out of the nest, Anthony still would pick fights with me, call me names, and put me down. It wasn't 24/7, but it was enough to bother me to the point of tears sometimes. I am usually a peacemaker, but after raising eight kids, I can get my temper going and try to give it back to him. But again, he held the power of being the breadwinner. I was contributing my time and my efforts, but I depended on him for money. Women today know better than to put themselves in this position, but I am of the old school, being 80 years of age, and Anthony is 82."

**Rosemary** added, "A few years ago, Anthony and I were grocery shopping together. We got into an argument in the grocery store, and he started yelling at me in public. He got all bent out of shape about something and took it out on me. We were near the meat section of the store, and he called me 'stupid' and told me that I 'didn't know what I was talking about.' He created quite a scene and then walked away from me as I was standing there red-faced and crying. A man who worked at the deli counter came over to me with a glass of water and a chair and asked if I needed anything else. He was so kind; I will never forget that day. I was so upset and embarrassed. Other women shoppers looked at me with pity. This was a low point for me because Anthony was taking his anger and frustrations out on me. Maybe because the kids were all out of the nest, I was the only one left to berate, criticize, and put down. But when you get to this age, you simply stay because you don't know what else to do. The only place I could go is to visit my kids, but they all have their own lives and jobs, and some have kids of their own. I don't suffer in silence because I have my sister and brother, my church group, and my sewing circle, and I volunteer at the Red Cross and the Visiting Nurses Association. I thank God for my kids and my women friends."

### Brenda and Jeff

**Brenda** reported, "I was married at age 20, had my first child at age 21, the second at age 22, and the third at age 25. This was the 1960s. There was a point in time when I had three children under the age of four. We moved around because Jeff was in the Army after college. I got married while in college between my junior and senior years. My former husband had been in ROTC in college and had to put his time in after college. He was obligated to go into the Army as a second lieutenant. I probably got married that summer because I felt like I would expire if I wasn't near him (laugh). He was a year older than I was, so that is why I interrupted my education a bit to go with him. We were facing the possibility of Jeff being sent to Vietnam. That colored my decision to stop school. Then the Army transferred us to Indiana. My oldest son was born at the hospital on an Army post in Indiana. He had surgery there for pyloric stenosis. Then, we moved to Maryland, and our daughter was born there. As I look back even then, there were incidents of verbal abuse by my husband and minor physical abuse. I question now, like many other people do, if any physical abuse is minor. However, none of them resulted in a trip to the hospital."

"Jeff drank in college, but so did everyone. Then, we moved from place to place with the Army, and then the drinking became more obvious. I must admit that at the time I was a good Catholic girl, and you consider marriage as being forever and try to have a positive attitude that everything is going to be wonderful and that things are going to change for the better. Well, it got worse, much worse. The physical abuse became more serious, and being a nurse, I was able to cover things up pretty well, and the verbal abuse was just abhorrent. Many people say that verbal abuse is the worst and leaves more scars. Your self-worth can be affected. I again was self-sufficient. I was so good at preventing the children from knowing what was going on with their father and how he treated me. I wanted to protect them from knowing. Although my oldest son once said to me shortly after he graduated from college, 'We know you have kept the family together.' There had also been financial problems. My former husband was spending money left and right. Sometimes the bills didn't get paid, and he was the one who was supposed to take care of the bills. That was his role in the family. I remember one time I went to the drug store and the manager there told me that our bill had not been paid in a couple of months. This was embarrassing, to say the least. He was in the Army for about three years and got out just before everyone was deployed to Vietnam. He got out to go back to school for his master's degree. The Army was a good experience, in that he had to behave better regarding drinking. The Army doesn't tolerate that stuff. He was an officer and was supposed to set a good example for his men. Then we moved to Albany for him to do a master's degree, and I took a position on the faculty there after a year or so. I had finished my BS degree in nursing by that time and was working in a hospital. Jeff was an extremely intelligent guy. He had graduated summa cum laude. He had a lot of talents, but like many alcoholics at the root of this was the fact that he was very insecure. On the other hand, I was just very capable, and I was juggling three kids and working. I think he resented me."

**Brenda** continued, "I remember being back in New York State before that to finish school because you couldn't change schools at that point when I just had to finish senior year. When I went back to school the children were 9 months and 20 months, as I recall. They were 11 months apart. I hadn't had the third one yet, my younger son. During that year, I remember being alone in the evenings after being in class or clinical all day. I would usually be home by about 3 PM, and I would get everything ready for the next day. I would get the kids' clothes ready and lay everything out. I would even get everything out for breakfast in case I had to leave early for the clinical. Jeff would be with the children until the babysitter arrived. He would go to work at 9 AM. But, while I was home at night, he was out. I was home studying, and he would go out. He said I would study better if he wasn't around, so he went out. He was out drinking and carousing. I could remember at the time feeling how nice it would be to have someone who cared about you and all that sort of stuff. I wished that our relationship was better. But here we already had these two children. It was a different time, and people thought differently. As I said, there was verbal as well as physical abuse. I can remember driving one time and being slapped across the face as I was driving. There was a broken tooth another time. I was good at covering up. I remember saying to someone that I had to go to the dentist because I tripped going up the stairs to the loft in the garage. Another time I remember going to a business meeting in Syracuse and the wives were invited. I wanted to cover up something with my eyes. I don't know if they were too red or bruised. So, the next day I wore sunglasses. There were outrageous demands about what I should do, what I should wear, and what I shouldn't wear. He was controlling me as much as he could. He had a strong sense of jealousy. I remember being berated as we went to a concert with two other couples. There were six of us in the car. I was berated because this very nice man was sitting next to me as if I planned it. This jealousy predominated. This couple's backyard backed up to our backyard. This man was so solicitous to everyone. I remember my neighbor and I said how nice it must be to have a husband like that. He was just so nice as was his wife. My former husband was just jealous of everything and anything."

As Jeff was accusing me of things, he was out having affairs, ongoing affairs. I knew about some of them because I would get phone calls from some of them telling me that he told them what a good person I was. There were many nights that he didn't come home. One time when this was going on I knew the address of the woman. The kids were very young, and I got the kids dressed in their snowsuits and we drove over there. I decided to do something about this. The kids stayed in the car. As I approached the apartment, I could hear his voice, and I knocked on the door and saw them. She had black lingerie on; I took off my wedding ring, and threw it at him. My biggest fear that day was that I had to leave the children in the car for about a minute and a half. Sometimes, he disappeared for days."

"I remember a few times when the kids had to step over him in the morning as he was passed out on the floor, to go out the door to school. In retrospect, I think 'Why didn't I do more?' But then, you have to think of it in terms of the times from the 1960s into the 1970s. I did my best, and he was just spending money on anything but the family. I remember my mother sending gifts from time to time. One time she sent sets of sheets for the children's beds, and I took them to the store and returned them for cash. I can remember shopping with my last $20, and it was at a point in time when sugar was very expensive. I happened to buy a sugar substitute at the time. It was called 'Sugar Twin.' I was doing a lot of baking at the time, especially making cookies for the children. I remember the children saying that the cookies didn't taste the same. I thought to myself, I wasted that money out of the $20. At that time, I would get my paycheck and I would turn it over to him. That's the way everyone did it back then. He did the finances. I got screwed right up until the time we divorced, which became final in 1989. He had managed to squirrel away things that I didn't know about. He had things hidden, and to this day he hasn't worked. He moved to Florida around 1987. He got married within six months of our divorce becoming final. He's still with her. I don't know the details of how they met or anything. He had this big wedding, and the three granddaughters were there. Everyone was there except me. He left me in 1985. I remember planning to drive my oldest son to college and had the car packed and was ready to go, and Jeff shows up at the last minute drunk and gets into the car. He refused to get out of the car. Somehow, I finally got him out of the car, probably because he was so drunk. I managed to put the three kids in the car, and off we drove. Somehow, he tracked us down at the motel and showed up. This was the kind of behavior he exhibited. I tried to create a life for my kids."

"Another time I remember being invited on a trip with other corporate wives and husbands; one year it was the Dominican Republic, and another year it was Aruba. We stayed at my mother's home on Long Island because we were flying out of JFK. Well, Jeff got up during the night and consumed an entire carafe of whiskey. I remember that the taxi was waiting, and he was trying to shave. Well, it was too bad that he didn't cut his throat. I hid this all from my mother. She was a smart woman and a good businesswoman, so she might have suspected something. I didn't want to burden her with knowing how things were. Why bother her with it; she couldn't do anything about it. We are all so stupid, us Catholics. Those nuns bent our minds. You didn't even tell your best friend about this bad, negative stuff. Also, at the time women were made to feel like they were responsible for the abuse. You know, like it was their fault. As the taxi driver was waiting, he said to me, 'What can I do to help?' And I remember saying, "Just be good to your children.' Also, 'The best thing a father can do for his children is to love their mother.' It is so simple and yet so profound. I tried to shield my children, but they are not stupid. Sometimes it was the tone of his voice even more than the words. Even before they can interpret words, they would hear that angry tone."

### Elena and Warren

**Elena** shared, "I met Warren when I was in high school. I was 17, and he was 19. We courted, had a long engagement, and then married in 1993. I loved him dearly, and I still do. He's the father of my daughter. I believe he has a mental illness, but he's never agreed to be evaluated. That's part of the issue when someone has not agreed to be diagnosed and treated. There was always underlying emotional abuse throughout our courtship, engagement, and marriage. He was my biggest fan and my worst enemy. Of course, you have good days and bad days, and the good days get you through the bad days. There were more bad days than good days. I was trying to stay in the marriage at least until our daughter went to college. Our daughter, Violet, is now 28 years old. When Violet was a senior in high school, I couldn't take it any longer, especially when he blamed me for the snow on the ground. I remember we were driving away, and he was pounding on the window of my car, blaming me for the snow, and I said I simply cannot do this anymore. Violet said, 'I don't blame you.' And on that day, I made plans to leave. I never really felt physically threatened, but I endured hours and hours and hours of being berated, just beaten down. He stayed home and didn't work. I wouldn't call him lazy; I think he was sick. I had more earning potential, so I returned to work six weeks after my c/s birth. I struggled with motherhood and working all three shifts in a week. I just finished a 16-hour double shift coming into Christmas Day, and this was Violet's first Christmas, and I had big plans. But I was physically exhausted, and my plans blew up in smoke. He sat me down on Christmas Eve and told me that I was a failure as a wife and a mother. There was absolutely nothing to celebrate. He continued to keep this main theme, and I knew there was trouble!"

"Warren stayed home while I worked. I worked some high-power jobs. Some weeks I was putting in about 70 hours per week trying to support the family. I enjoyed what I did, but he didn't see this as a sacrifice. He saw him staying home as a sacrifice. He took care of the baby. He insists that I ruined his chance of becoming a teacher because of my work schedule. He accused me of ruining his life. He said that I am nothing without him, and everything that I accomplished in my life was because of him. When I got my master's degree, I graduated with a 3.98 GPA, and on the ride home from the graduation he told me that it was his degree."

**Elena** added, "I sing in the choir at church, and I am very involved with that. I do all the Masses on Sunday mornings. That is my spiritual food, and I guess because I am good at that and I take pride in that, he said that I was being selfish. Every Sunday he tried to make me feel bad that I was gone on Sunday mornings. Everything good in my life, he saw as selfish. He tried to attack everything good for me. He said all my accomplishments were on his back; I could not have done anything without him. I mean there were hours and hours and hours of yelling. He said that my work was ruining the family, but I was the only one working. Someone had to work, so I'm not sure what else I could have done. When I was home, the tension was high. I felt bad for my daughter, especially as she got older. When I had a few days off I would try to do the things I wanted to do with her. I wished I could do this all along, but I had to work. I tried to make dinner one night and the stove broke, but he refused to have anyone come in and fix it. Yet, I was a failure as a wife because I didn't have a stove to cook on. He would say, just because you have cooked a few meals doesn't make you a good wife. I heard that several times. I got this message from him all my adult life."

**Elena** reported, "I finally got out on March 1, 2011. I thought I was over it. But sometimes I think I'm not completely over the whole thing. I am still responsible for him financially. It was February 27 or 28 when he called me out of the church and there was snow on the ground. He had to take our daughter to Massachusetts for some softball thing. The car he was driving slipped on our very long driveway, and so he called me to say that I must come and get Violet and take her where she needs to go. He blamed it on me that he got his car stuck in the driveway. I was stunned, and I started backing my car down the driveway. Violet got in my car, and he kept banging on the window of my car yelling that I ruined his life. I got on the road and said to myself, 'I just can't do this anymore.' Violet was 17 at this point, the same age I was when I started dating her father. I said to her, 'I'll leave.' And she said, 'I don't blame you.' The house that we lived in was right next to his father's house. So, Violet stayed with her father in our family home, and I left and stayed with a friend. Also, I didn't want to take Violet out of her school system, away from her friends. My leaving was fuel for his fire. I abandoned the family in his eyes. But I had to get out for myself. It's funny because I still did the grocery shopping for all of us. I paid all the bills. And I was staying with a friend who lived an hour away. Violet even told me that it was better this way. She said, 'It's not so tense at home.' She was able to complete her senior year living at home. I moved her into college and started my separate relationship with her. I would visit her weekly up in Massachusetts."

**Elena** stated, "There are two things: I wanted to be respectful of her father. She saw what she saw, and I couldn't do much about that. She didn't need to hear me say that her dad was abusive. He would take a lot of time to say to her, 'Where is your mom now? She's not with you.' He did his best to poison her mind against me. And it worked to a certain extent. Just now, over the last few years, Violet has concluded that maybe I wasn't that bad after all. It has taken her several years to realize that I did what I had to do. But still, I abandoned the family. I would be working on the weekend to pay for life for all of us, and he'd say, 'Where's your mother?' So, Violet grew up thinking that I was never around. She had a boyfriend who knew me well, and she would say certain things, and he'd say, 'Now hold on just a minute. Do you think maybe how you think you grew up is somehow skewed based on your mother working to support the family?' Violet has changed her thinking a bit. He knew the truth because he knew both of us. He saw my dedication to my kid. I'm trying to make up for the lost time, but I'll drop anything to go to her or to do something for her, or to just be with her. It's not a guilty conscience. I couldn't be there as much as I would have liked to through the years. She heard that I 'screwed her dad' with the divorce settlement. I paid him alimony and lost financially. And I continue to lose financially. I still support him financially, and he says that he couldn't work because my career took precedence. He stayed home to raise Violet. He still didn't work, and to this day, he still doesn't work. He still says everything was my fault."

"He destroyed my self-esteem, and my confidence, and made me question my abilities. I guess deep in my heart I believed all the awful things he said to me. I could still cry about all of this. I have to say that he shattered the way I thought about myself. I guess to some extent all the horrible things he said about me got to me. I had a really hard time."

"We were together for 27 years, and I heard negative things about myself for at least 25 of the 27 years. He did a lot of damage. We did go to marriage counseling after I left. He said I was keeping the finances from him. The marriage counselor was hearing his side of the story and I felt DONE. There was nothing anyone could say or do to change my mind. He said his piece, and I said, 'Does anyone want to know what I think?' I made my feelings known, and this was our third session. Well, he was spitting mad, and he started screaming. I had to hear all the stuff over again that I had been hearing for so many years. It came flying out of his mouth in front of the marriage counselor. The marriage counselor would say, 'Whoa, whoa, whoa, hold on a minute, that's not fair.' He went on about how I ruined his life, our daughter's life, and his father's life. He just kept yelling and could not control himself. The marriage counselor could not control him either. He kept spitting and sputtering, and I said to the marriage counselor, 'This is what I have been putting up with for so many years, almost our entire marriage and I've had enough." I stood up and said, "I am not going to put up with this anymore," and the marriage counselor said, 'I think that's a good idea.' He truly believes that I ruined his life, and I do feel bad about that. The underlying problem is that there is a mental illness involved that he is not willing to address. I mean let's face it, our daughter is grown, and we've been divorced for nine years, and he still receives a weekly check from me, and he has not made any effort to go to work or go back to school. He's never been able to get it together because he is sick. He simply wants to blame me and not his illness."

### Maureen and Paul

**Maureen** reported, "I had been living with my three teenagers in the house. It certainly kept life interesting after my divorce. As the kids one by one left home for college, I started to date again. I never seemed to have trouble meeting interesting men, and they were almost always well-educated. I guess the fact that I taught at a university helped. Yet, I didn't meet them at work. I met them at conferences or through research endeavors or colleagues or friends. I began dating Paul, and he had a Ph.D. from Yale University. He seemed to be well-regarded in the intellectual community. Initially, I did not see any 'red flags' with this man."

"However, Paul was not always honest about some of the elements of his life, and it took me four years in this relationship to find out that he had been married three times. I don't know why he could not be honest with me about his past relationships. I think he had at least seven or nine significant relationships before me, and he married at least three of them. I suspect it might have even been four marriages. Over time, he became more and more controlling. He wanted to know where I was at all times and who I was with. At first, I thought he was being protective, but later I realized that he was controlling. He also became verbally abusive when he didn't get what he wanted or I didn't say the right thing. I thought to myself, 'Why do I always meet controlling men like the husband I divorced years ago? Why do these men always lie so much? Are they afraid I'll run for the hills because they were previously married? Are they all looking for someone they can dominate?' Well, the verbal abuse and controlling behavior caused me to break off the relationship after four years. I had enough of his lies, control, and bad behavior. This was not my first rodeo."

### Beatrice and Brett

**Beatrice** stated, "I went back into my journal to be able to accurately tell you about my experience with my first husband. I was married to Brett for seven years, and we had one son together. I married him after college and traveled a bit. I was 25 years old. It was a 6-month whirlwind romance. He wanted to get married right away. During our marriage, he tried to control me. The verbal and emotional abuse was not constant; it was intermittent. There was no hitting or shoving, but I was called 'a selfish bitch' many, many times during those seven years. Why did I stay with him? I probably stayed because of my strong religious upbringing. I come from a large family of seven children. Marriage was supposed to be forever."

"I must tell you that I have worked hard to learn to forgive myself for staying with him. It was not a good situation for my son or myself. It has been a life-long challenge to overcome the blow to my self-esteem.' I had some psychiatric training in school, but that was with patients who were quite mentally ill and were hospitalized or institutionalized. My husband was not one of them. However, I came to realize that he had severe anger management problems and was very narcissistic. Most of the time, I walked on eggshells whenever we were together. I grew to be afraid of his temper. I didn't know how things were going to turn out for my son and me. I realized that this was no way to live. I kept hoping things would improve, but they never did."

"For seven years, I minimalized his bad behavior in my mind. I felt trapped. However, I went into marriage thinking that it would be forever. He was controlling, very hurtful, and talked to me in a very demeaning way. My self-esteem hit rock bottom. I almost can't put into words how hurtful this experience was for me. To be honest, He shattered my heart, and the remaining scar has never completely healed."

### Taryn and Chuck

**Taryn** shared, "I did not realize I was in an abusive marriage until after our son was born. When Chuck and I were dating, there was no emotional or verbal abuse. Chuck was always very self-centered and wanted my full attention. Although he loved our son and was a good father, he lacked patience at times and seemed jealous of my attention to the baby. However, what was I to do? Babies and little kids need their mother's attention. I tried to be a good wife and mother, but it was never enough for Chuck after the birth. With each passing month, he seemed to grow impatient with me and find fault with almost everything I did. He thought I relied too much on my parents, but they lived across town and were retired. Eli was their first grandchild, and they were thrilled to see him regularly."

**Taryn** continued, "Pretty soon the arguments between me and Chuck got more frequent. He thought he was my intellectual superior because he had a master's degree and I only went to junior college. I was content to be an executive secretary and administrative assistant. I was good at my job and liked the company I worked for. I worked with a great bunch of people and had a wonderful boss. Chuck had an elitist attitude and felt entitled to things. He was materialistic and always had to have the best of everything. He was never content with having a nice house, wife, and son."

**Taryn** added, "When Eli was about two years old, Chuck started punching me in the arm when he was angry. He would yell at me, which he had done in the past. But now, he would give me a little punch in the arm, too. This escalated over the next two years, and both of my arms had bruises on them. He never really beat me up; there were no black eyes or bloody lips. I started wearing long-sleeved shirts, blouses, and sweaters so no one would see the bruises. It wasn't like I got a new bruise every day, but when Chuck would get mad at me or have a bad day at work or if Eli was getting on his nerves, he would talk very harshly, call me names, and punch me in the arm. He'd call me 'stupid' or say that I was doing this wrong or that wrong. He belittled me for not going to a four-year college and said that he hoped that Eli inherited his brains because I didn't have any. He put me down and deflated my ego to the extent that I felt worthless, that I wasn't good at anything."

"I remember my mother asking me why I was wearing a long-sleeved shirt in the summer when it was over 90 degrees outside. I made up a bunch of excuses. I said things like the air conditioning bothered me and I didn't like the way my arms looked in a tank top. I also said I was afraid of bug bites and didn't want to get sunburned. Chuck never punched me in front of anyone else, even Eli. We tended to have our 'arguments' when Eli was asleep. I hid everything from my parents, too."

**Taryn** concluded, "I finally asked Chuck for a divorce because I didn't want to live this way anymore. I was also afraid that he'd start punching Eli. My parents had a wonderful, loving marriage, and I knew I would be better off without Chuck. I grew to dislike him and realized that I made a mistake marrying him. His 'charm' had worn off big time. He was a different person before I married him, but maybe that was all an act. Once he got me locked into a relationship as a wife and mother, he treated me more like a possession or a servant. I knew I didn't want to raise Eli in this environment, and I wanted out. I suspect that Chuck may have been involved with other women, especially when he went on a business trip, but I have no real proof, just a suspicion. I think my parents tolerated Chuck, but there was no love lost between them, if you know what I mean. They could see that I was not happy with him; I was always walking on a tightrope, waiting to be reprimanded for making another mistake. Eli and I are much happier, and we live with my parents. Chuck pays child support but no alimony. We worked out a schedule for him to see Eli, and that is going well. Chuck usually takes Eli to sporting events."

### Susan and Scott

**Susan** reported, "We met in an executive training program for a large global company after graduate school. Our attraction to each other was immediate. I thought that Scott was charming, handsome, and smart. He told me that he came from a very wealthy family. Basically, he took my breath away. I come from a middle-class family and grew up in a farming community in Pennsylvania. I was an 'A' student in high school, graduated with honors from college, and did well in graduate school. I have always been close to my family and have had a lot of friends. I love people!"

**Susan** continued, "We got married after we completed the executive training program. Scott worked in marketing, and I worked in human relations at different but nearby facilities for the same company. I had an unplanned pregnancy after being married for a year. I was surprised but accepted the wonderful news. I have always dreamed of having three or four children. Conversely, Scott was in a state of shock about the pregnancy. He simply was not ready for it. He had always said that 'money would never be a problem' but did not share my enthusiasm for parenthood. I worked up until I went into labor and gave birth to a healthy 8-pound, 10-ounce baby girl. We named her Julie-Ann."

**Susan** added, "Scott would not get up with the baby in the middle of the night or change diapers. Eight hours of uninterrupted sleep was a priority for him. So, I often slept in the nursery with the baby. I took a six-month maternity leave, breastfed, and thoroughly enjoyed motherhood. I then extended my time off to nine months to be home with Julie-Ann. As I prepared to return to work, I found out that I was pregnant again. I had not had a period and was still breastfeeding so I didn't think I could get pregnant so easily. I accepted the reality of the situation and thought it would be okay to have close siblings. I thought it would be nice for the kids to be close in age. However, I was stunned by Scott's reaction to the second pregnancy; he was outraged. He was angry and sullen, and told me that I was a 'stupid female.' He said, 'How could you let this happen again?' He told me that I was 'a major fuck-up.' He was furious and blamed me for 'not thinking and being careless.' I was so hurt by his reaction. I thought he would calm down, but he didn't. He had been distant and detached even before Julie Ann was born, but now his behavior was worse. He was mean, cruel, and verbally abusive. He behaved like a spoiled brat. I thought, 'Was this the same man I married?'

**Susan** reported, "Our relationship deteriorated over the next few months. I decided not to return to work because finances were not a problem. Scott had a trust fund and would inherit everything from his parents because he was an only child. Scott called me a 'house frau' and told me that I was 'wasting my entire education' by staying home. Scott did not accompany me to prenatal visits but instead immersed himself in work."

**Susan** stated, "His recreation was not spending time with me and Julie-Ann, it was doing stuff with his guy friends who did not have kids. He played basketball, golf, and tennis. I did 90% of the household chores as well as all of the childcare. Scott would do the bulk of the grocery shopping on Sunday afternoons."

**Susan** confided that Scott threatened not to be present at the birth of their second child. She said that he was still angry and detached. She also said that their verbal communication was tense and awkward under the circumstances. She shared that he said that he 'had enough.'"

**Susan** recalled, "Much to my surprise, Scott was present at the birth of our second daughter, Jody-Lynn, who weighed in at nine pounds two ounces. Scott 'went through the motions' at the hospital, but he was not happy. He would have preferred to have a son instead of another daughter, but ultimately, he did not want kids in his life or at least not as a 34-year-old executive. Scott was an only child and had no exposure to babies or young children."

"Within six months after the birth of Jody-Lynn, Scott told me that he 'wanted out.' He said that he would always provide for the girls financially, but that this was not the life he envisioned for himself. He didn't want the responsibilities of being a husband and father. Scott's announcement made me feel crushed and abandoned. Yet, I was tired of the lack of emotional support, the name-calling, the anger, the arguing, and the daily unpleasantness. We obtained a divorce, and Scott kept his financial obligations. I am happier apart from Scott and not having to listen to him putting me down, criticizing me, yelling at me, and treating me like a servant."

### Barbara and Jay

**Barbara** stated, "My husband was only 58 when he died from chronic alcoholism and heart failure. I was only 49. He was a social drinker when we got married, and I occasionally had a cocktail with him. I had no idea how much he drank in the early years of our marriage, but I suspect he drank some when I was not home. He was very good at holding his liquor. He never slurred his words or acted as if he had too much to drink. He went to work every day and was on time for appointments, his grooming standards were impeccable, and he never in the first ten years of our marriage appeared like he had a drinking problem. We had fun, traveled, entertained, and prospered in the first ten years of our marriage."

"Jay retired from his civil service government job at about the time of our tenth wedding anniversary. I noticed some changes after his retirement. He put on about 20 pounds, started taking afternoon naps, seemed kind of apathetic, had no hobbies to keep him busy, and was only making a half-hearted attempt to find a job in the non-government sector. Meanwhile, my career was thriving. He always handled paying the bills. He was always right on time, but now I noticed we started to get some late notices, even though we had plenty of money in our account. He had always been on top of our finances until he retired. I think he was depressed now that I look back, but he wanted to retire after 20 years in civil service. It was his choice, not forced retirement. His boss was a younger man whom he didn't always get along with. His boss was ambitious but a decent guy. My husband didn't hate him, but I think he resented this man and his many accomplishments."

**Barbara** continued, "At about our tenth anniversary, I started to notice these changes. When I confronted Jay about late bill notices, he got defensive, but he usually paid them after I nagged him. Then I noticed that he was having a drink or two right after lunch and then taking a nap. I'd come home from my office, and he'd be sound asleep. He'd curse me out if I woke him up. He'd curse me out if I asked about his job hunting, most of which he did over the phone or through the mail. He'd wear the same shorts and golf shirt for three or four days at a time. He'd shave about every other day. He seemed angry at me all the time and angry at the world. I guess he was depressed, but I didn't ponder that at the time, I thought he was just being lazy and self-indulgent. I started to feel that he resented my happiness in my work, my promotions, and my network of friends and colleagues."

**Barbara** added, "One time I was preparing leftovers rather than cooking a fresh meal, and he threw a plate of spaghetti at me and went across the street and had dinner with our neighbors. Another time he was supposed to pick me up at the airport, and he kept me waiting for him for three hours. This was before cell phones, so I was stuck because he didn't answer the house phone. Another time he took me out for dinner, saying he 'wanted to talk about something.' He proceeded to tell me that a neighbor was going to tell me that he 'came on to his wife.' Jay said it was just an 'innocent, friendly invitation to come over for a drink' since both of their spouses were away. I got mad and walked out of the restaurant before the meal came, and I walked three miles to our house. It was supposed to be my birthday dinner."

"Jay was never physically abusive, but he was emotionally abusive. When he was angry or in a bad mood, he would call me names or say negative things about my family. He was jealous of my career success instead of being happy for me or appreciative. He had a mean streak when he was drinking."

### Marjorie and Tad

**Marjorie** stated, "I knew Tad had a temper when I married him. He was a football player in college and was known for being tough, forceful, and brutal on the field. However, he was never that way with me while dating. He was fun-loving, considerate, and romantic. We married after graduating from a large mid-western university."

According to Marjorie, "We decided to delay starting a family so that we could both become established in our careers and buy a house. After being married for five years and setting up a nice home, I started talking with Tad about planning for a baby. I sensed that Tad was not ready to start a family. It didn't happen overnight, but slowly and surely, I started to realize that Tad and I were on different wavelengths. He was obsessed with his job in commercial real estate. He liked wining and dining and meeting rich, influential people. Over time I became somewhat invisible to Tad. I loved my job as a preschool teacher and felt that I was good at it. Tad never asked me about my work, whereas I always listened to his stories about business deals and the big wigs he interacted with regularly."

**Marjorie** reported, "Tad built a separate world apart from me. He became short-tempered every time I brought up the subject of starting a family. When a business deal went south, he would explode and punch the wall to the extent that I always got a repairman in when Tad was on a business trip to fix the latest hole in the wall. Tad accused me of 'being in a child's world' and 'not keeping up with the financial world of wheeling and dealing.' I felt that Tad looked down on me and did not consider me his equal partner. Sometimes he would call me 'dumb' and tell me that I was not financially astute. The things he used to like about me and the fun times we had in the past simply went out the window."

**Marjorie** continued, "I could not prove that Tad cheated on me with other women from the business world, but I would not be surprised if he did. Tad's ego grew with every successful business deal, and he came to enjoy the nicer things in life. I constantly questioned myself thinking, 'Is this the same man I married?'

**Marjorie** added, "Tad stopped involving me in his life except when he wanted sex. We continued to live together unhappily. He came home for dinner about 50% of the time if he didn't have a business dinner or a handball game with a friend at the gym. He always played football with a group of college friends and business associates on Saturday mornings. Tad was religious about his Saturday morning football games. When I suggested marriage counseling, Tad blew up. He yelled at me and forcefully backed me up to the wall. His behavior frightened me because he was full of rage. I was terrified. Here he is, this big guy and I'm 5'4" and 120 pounds. He never hit me, but he shoved me several times. I also lived in fear that he'd punch me in the face like he'd punch the wall in our house. I grew to be afraid of my husband. When life did not go his way, he'd take it out on me by yelling, cursing, and punching the wall."

**Marjorie** continued, "To make a long story short, I moved out of our house when Tad was on a business trip. I stayed with my best friend from college for three months until I found an apartment of my own. Subsequently, I divorced Tad, and he did not contest it. We both realized that we had grown apart, and he chose his flashy business career over our marriage and a possible family in the future. The judge advised Tad to get help and enroll in an anger management program. I don't know if he ever did. His inflated ego and macho demeanor may have kept him from getting the help he needs."

**Marjorie** concluded, "In the four years since I left Tad, I have adopted two children and built a wonderful life for the three of us. It is such a relief not to be afraid of an angry, abusive husband anymore. I feel lucky to have escaped because many women don't have the happy ending that I have. I feel blessed."

The aforementioned narratives supply testimony to the realization of an abusive relationship. The behavioral features of the marital relationships changed with these couples, and a new dynamic emerged which included anger, control, emotional abuse, and sometimes physical harm. There were some common elements in all the women's stories.

Many women talked about emotional trauma. This type of trauma was more prevalent than physical trauma. It can stay with a person for the rest of their life. Specifically, emotional trauma is the result of events or experiences that can leave a person feeling upset, unsafe, fearful, and often helpless. It can result from a single event or be part of an ongoing situation or circumstances, such as chronic abuse, discrimination, harassment, bullying, or humiliation.

People with PTSD can have intense disturbing feelings and thoughts related to the problematic experience. These upsetting feelings and thoughts can last long after the traumatic experience has ended. People may relive the event or experience it through flashbacks and nightmares; they may feel sadness, fear, or anger. They may feel detached or estranged from others, including family and friends.

Trauma is an emotional response to a terrible event like a serious motor vehicle accident, a mugging, or a rape. The event might be a natural disaster like an earthquake or a wartime ambush or explosion. It could also be an awful experience such as being served with divorce papers at work, being slapped in the face by a significant other, having to confront a cheating husband, dealing with the sudden loss of a close friend to death, or living with continual domestic abuse.

### Theme: Fear of Him; Threats, Control, Pain, and Isolation

Women told of fear of their abuser. There were frightening threats, strict control and manipulation, emotional pain, and enforced isolation. Some experienced physical violence as well. They were sleeping with the enemy. The following quotations illustrate their lived experience:

**Sabrina**: "I was afraid for myself and my daughter. Antonio's temper would sometimes explode. One time he pulled a barrette out of my hair, another time he ripped my nightgown right off me. Another time I questioned him about a woman, and he didn't like it, and in a fit of anger, he threw me across the room, and I broke my wrist. My wrist bone came through the skin. He left the house, and I had to drive myself to the hospital with my three-year-old daughter. They questioned me at the hospital and asked me how this happened. I lied and said that I tripped and fell. To this day, I don't know why I lied."

**Joanne**: "Theo engaged in gaslighting and stonewalling to undermine me. He had an elitist attitude and probably delusions of grandeur because he considered himself an expert on a plethora of things. It almost made me laugh when he would espouse being an expert on parenting with basically no experience. I think because he was a lawyer, he considered himself superior to the rest of us mortals. What bothered me the most was the way he tried to exert control over me. Everything was about control, about him approving what I did, where I went, what I fed June, and whom June played with. I felt like a prisoner in my own home. Theo wanted me to ask for permission to do anything, whether it was to meet with my mother's group or take June to the park. He was somewhat controlling before June was born, but things got a hundred times worse when we became parents. He would criticize almost everything I did, and during an angry tirade, he would occasionally throw something at me. This was usually after June was asleep. He was a loving and interested father to June. It was me that was the subject of his wrath. He wanted me to always ask for permission to go somewhere or to do something.

He started being even more controlling at one point with domestic chores, saying that I couldn't load the dishwasher because I did it wrong. I was forbidden to use or clean the steak knives because I was scratching and bending them. He also said I bought groceries that we didn't need and forgot to get the ones that we did need. He did not complain about these things when we were first married. I wondered, 'What had changed?' He drove my self-esteem into the ground. But I was determined not to leave until June went off to college."

**Marcella**: "The emotional abuse was something I will never forget. The level of control was frightening. I had never experienced anything like this in my life. Wyatt was not this way when we were dating in college. After saying our wedding vows, it was like he took ownership of me. I remember that he wouldn't let me fly home to be a bridesmaid at the wedding of my best friend from high school. My widowed mother was paying for my ticket because she was also going to the wedding. Mom wanted me to visit her for the week. Wyatt said that I could not go because it was my place to be with him since I was his wife. It broke my heart that I couldn't attend Patrice's wedding. In addition, my mother was very disappointed, too. It became clear to me over time that Wyatt didn't truly care about how I felt or my mother for that matter. He wanted to make all the decisions in our marriage, always being in the driver's seat. What I thought would be an equal partnership turned out to be the opposite. Many times, to keep the peace, I would go along with what he wanted because his temper frightened me. I would go out of my way to please him. I would cook his favorite meals, entertain his friends, stay within the budget, keep the apartment clean, iron his shirts, do all the laundry and grocery shopping, and always say 'yes' to sex even if I was tired from work. When I look back on those years, I see myself as a robot or like the old movie *The Stepford Wives*."

Wyatt acted so miserably when he was in graduate school that I would do almost anything to cheer him up. I wanted to try to get the old Wyatt back, the man I married. But that Wyatt was long gone. I wonder if that Wyatt ever really existed because I never saw him again after our wedding. He trapped me; he held me hostage. To this day, I have no idea how he fooled me so easily. Now, when I look back on my college years and the years we were married, I consider it such a waste of my precious time. He robbed me of my youth and innocence. I believe that being betrayed by the person you love is the cruelest act because it shatters your heart, breaks your spirit, and tears apart your inner core of being. You are never completely healed because the remaining scar will always be there."

**Bethany**: "Jordan whittled away at my self-esteem. He tried to cut me off from my family and friends. He had a sexual addiction and would demand sex. I remember lying there sometimes thinking that this was marital rape. Jordan found fault with everything I did around our home. He berated everything I did, whether it was the meals I prepared or the way I ironed his shirts. Whatever I did, it was just never good enough."

**Andrea**: "I hated for my kids to be hit with a belt when they didn't deserve it. I tried to protect them and got hit also. When Mike was drinking, he had a short fuse at home. I bore the brunt of it at times with the harsh language, flared temper, and the occasional leather belt. I tried to keep peace in the house, but sometimes things got out of hand. I didn't want the kids to be afraid of their father. But they couldn't help being afraid; I was afraid. I tried to deny reality and cover up Mike's bad behavior. I made excuses for him. Down deep, I knew he was a good man when he was not drinking. When he died of a heart attack, it was almost a relief. But I still loved him, and I know the kids loved him too."

**Rosemary**: "Many people probably wonder why I have stayed with Anthony for so many years. With eight kids I felt like I had to stick it out. I made those marriage vows, you know. I grew up at a time when people didn't get divorced. I learned to steer clear when Anthony was in a bad mood. I avoided him when I could see that he was getting annoyed or frustrated. But sometimes he brought me to my knees with insults, criticism, and name-calling. Growing up in our house was not easy for any of our eight kids. I think they all went off to college or the military service as quickly as they could. There was always this underlying tension in our house."

**Brenda:** "In retrospect, I got married to Jeff because I felt like I couldn't live without him. He was a year ahead of me in college, so I interrupted my education to marry him. What a mistake that was. Before I knew it, we had two babies and then later a third. Life was stressful. In time, I found out that Jeff was unfaithful and liked his alcohol. When I was studying to finish my degree, he was out sleeping around and drinking. I sheltered the kids as much as I could, but they were not blind. Jeff was both mentally and physically abusive. There was an occasional slap, but most of the abuse was verbal and behavioral. Initially, I believed that marriage was forever, but it got worse, much worse. The verbal abuse was awful, and it left scars. My self-worth was diminished. Jeff was very intelligent, but like many alcoholics, at the root of this was the fact that he was insecure. My positive attitude and capabilities bothered him, and I was working and juggling three kids. He had a jealous streak."

**Elena**: "I endured hours and hours and hours of being berated, just beaten down. Warren told me over and over that I was a failure as a wife and mother. He blamed me for everything. He accused me of not being there enough for him and Violet, yet someone had to work to pay the mortgage and put food on the table. I still don't know what I could have done differently to support the three of us. I did the best I could, but it was never good enough for Warren. He attacked and criticized everything good in my life, like singing in the church choir. When we were in the house together, tension was high. I finally got out in 2011, but I'm still not over the whole thing. I have flashbacks and nightmares."

**Maureen**: "Paul was not honest about a lot of things. He had a way of evading the truth, changing the subject, or downright lying. He was well-educated, charming, witty, and fun. Over time, he became more and more controlling and verbally abusive. He wanted to know where I was at all times and who I was with. He brought negativity into my life. I realized that I could not trust Paul to be honest, considerate, kind, and to treat me the way I should be treated with respect. There is a lot more verbal abuse around than most people realize. Most women simply take it, especially if they share kids with the man or are not financially independent. They put up with controlling behaviors, threats, and put-downs, and their self-esteem ends up in the toilet. No woman should have to put up with someone like Paul, and I almost married him. His actions caused me to end the relationship. I saved myself."

**Beatrice**: "We were married for seven years. The control and verbal abuse grew over time. He called me a 'selfish bitch' and a slew of other names. He talked to me in a very demeaning way and made very hurtful comments that I will never forget. I came from a big, loving family and had never been exposed to anything like this. He had major anger management problems and was very self-absorbed. I grew to have a victim mentality, and I didn't like that one bit, but I was certainly a victim. I was afraid, and I needed to protect my son."

She continued, "Bart would yell at me and berate me in front of our son. He referred to me as 'undereducated,' didn't like the way I folded the laundry, and complained about my cooking. He would not do this in front of other people; it only happened when we were alone, but he did not shield our son. His treatment of me was a blow to my self-esteem. A few times he tried to keep me from seeing my family. I remember packing the car to take our son, Billy, with me to a family cookout, and Bart threw the car seat at me as I was in the process of putting it in the car. He said, 'You're not taking Billy,' and I said, 'Yes, I am.' Then he yelled, 'Go see your miserable family.' He also warned me not to tell anyone what had transpired."

"Bart had come from an abusive family. He threatened that if I divorced him, he would kill himself. He was seven years older than me. I was afraid that if I didn't get out of the marriage, Billy would grow up to be like his father. Bart would get in a rage and say things to me like, 'I will impoverish you.' It was not a good situation for me, and I wanted to protect Billy."

**Taryn**: "The abuse started after our son, Eli, was born. Although Chuck loved Eli and was a good father, he lacked patience and seemed jealous of my attention to the baby. I tried to be a good wife and mother, but it was never enough for Chuck. He found fault with almost everything I did. He also thought I relied on my parents too much. My parents loved to babysit and helped us out when we had to go to a business dinner. Chuck always wanted the best of everything and was never satisfied. He never really beat me up; there were no black eyes or bloody lips. But there were almost always bruises on my arms. I was embarrassed and ashamed. Chuck would get mad at me a lot or punch me when he had a bad day at work. He'd call me a 'moron' or say that I was doing this wrong or that wrong. He belittled me for not going to a four-year college. He said hurtful things, mocked me, and put me down. I didn't want to continue living this way, so I finally got up enough nerve to ask Chuck for a divorce. I was also afraid that he might start punching Eli as he got older."

**Susan**: "I had two unplanned pregnancies which set my husband into a tailspin. He was angry and didn't want the responsibilities of parenthood at this point in his life. He was furious at me for 'letting this happen.' I didn't plan to get pregnant this early in our marriage, but I accepted it. I come from a warm, loving family and had hoped to have three or four children in the future. I was incredulous at Scott's temper tantrums, self-centeredness, and immaturity. This was not the man I thought I married. He threatened me and tried to control me. He was mean and cruel. I was frightened by his angry outbursts. He behaved so badly, and I felt betrayed and abandoned. He turned his back on me and our two daughters. He provides for the girls financially as promised."

**Barbara**: "When Jay retired, he became lazy and started to drink alcohol more often. He was a nasty drunk. He was inconsiderate of me, talked harshly to me, paid bills late, refused to drive me to the bus stop on very cold mornings, criticized some of the meals I made, and was generally mean-spirited. Before retirement, I would say that he was a 'functioning alcoholic.' When he was agitated, he would call me names, curse at me, yell at me, berate me, and upset me greatly with his behavior. Jay was a smart man with an MBA, who always insisted on doing our taxes and always submitted them on time. Well, once he retired, he was late filing our taxes three years in a row, and we had to pay substantial penalties. It was hard to tell if this behavior was from excessive drinking, laziness, or maybe depression. He lied to me each year and said he filed on time when he didn't. I also think he was jealous of my accomplishments and the fact that I was still working. His situation saddened me because he was not at all like this when we got married 16 years before. When he died of a heart attack, I was relieved."

**Marjorie**: "Our relationship had deteriorated while I waited to start a family. He became easily angered, frustrated, and bored. He only paid attention to me when he wanted to have sex. He was a controlling and bossy husband. When a business deal did not turn out the way he wanted it to, he would put his fist through the wall. This frightened me. I was never exposed to violent behavior. I kept thinking, 'What will I do if he starts hitting or punching me?' To make a long story short, I divorced Tad. Soon after, I adopted two children who are the 'lights of my life.'"

Fear was the mainstay of this theme. Women were on edge not knowing what to expect each day. They feared not only for their safety but for that of their children as well. Life was a rollercoaster some endured for years. Any of these women could have become a homicide statistic if things had escalated. None of the women in this study mentioned having to get a restraining order for police protection. They were fortunate because 13 of them left the abusive relationship. The woman who remained was in her 80s with eight grown children with whom she is close.

We have all heard the phrase, "time heals all wounds." However, in reviewing the interview transcripts of the 14 women in this study, that is not necessarily true. Several women in the research study highlighted in this book commented about their emotional scars. They mentioned having a broken heart, shattered dreams, flashbacks, and nightmares. They described fear, diminished self-esteem, betrayal, abandonment, and the emotional trauma that accompanies abuse. Some talked about being punched, slapped, shoved, and backed up to the wall. Fortunately, none of the women were stabbed, shot, or choked. Perhaps, they were the lucky ones.

### Theme: Accepting Support; Grabbing the Life Preserver

Women collectively applauded their support systems for making survival possible. Family, friends, and co-workers made a difference in these women's lives. Most were open to sharing details of their abuse with trusted family and friends. Their words speak to accepting support.

**Sabrina**: "My mom had written me a card and she didn't know the details because I had never shared them. I didn't want her to worry about me and my daughter. But she said in her card if you want to come home, take a plane. I think she had the mother's intuition because I never said that Antonio was abusive. I think she could tell. Her card said, 'We support you.'"

**Joanne**: "My family and friends are happy for me. No one blames me for leaving Theo and getting a divorce. The people in my life saw Theo's controlling behavior even when I tried to cover it up. They saw a change in me when I lost my strong sense of self. They saw me walk on eggshells, asking permission to do this or that, becoming overwhelmed with self-doubt, and trying to cover up Theo's bad behavior. With the support of family and friends, I divorced Theo. Now, I once again appreciate the beauty of nature, the wisdom of the elderly, and the wonderment of children. I joined a support group at church and had somewhat of a spiritual renewal. I always prayed for a good outcome for June and me. She went off to college and we are still very close. June says that she sees a much happier Mom now; I tried so hard for her not to see the cruel and abusive treatment that I endured at the hand of her father."

**Marcella**: "Although I shielded my family and friends from knowing the extent of the abuse, I finally had to tell them when I was moving out of the apartment I shared with Wyatt. Even though I still loved Wyatt, he held me down in so many ways. He was a very needy man. He always wanted his ego stroked, to be waited on, and to be coddled when he was in a bad mood. I bent over backward to please him, but I never did. I was his caregiver, his mistress, his cheerleader, and his devoted wife, but it was never enough. I was a prisoner in my own home. I was used and abused. I felt safer at work than at home. My mother came to visit when she realized how bad things were. She and my friends helped me move out. Mom admitted that Wyatt fooled her, too. He was not the person she thought he was. Friends were surprised, dumbfounded, outraged, disappointed, and saddened. People wondered how I managed to suffer in silence for so long. I was heart-broken, embarrassed, ashamed, and lost. I felt betrayed, lied to, and abandoned. I was afraid of Wyatt and the power he had. Yet, I knew that my wonderful family and support-ive friends would not let me starve. Plus, I had a job. But I needed my car for work, and he threatened to take it away from me. He treated me despicably, simply horribly, and I put up with it. That was a big mistake on my part, but I didn't know what else to do. He was my college sweetheart, and I wasted 11 years in the relationship."

**Bethany**: "I have three wonderful kids who kept me going. I also have caring parents and a close-knit band of siblings. My big extended family is friendly and fun-loving, too. I am blessed. Then, I have several friends from grad school and others from work whom I can depend on. I needed everyone to help me come to terms with my situation and finally leave Jordan. I stayed too long under the circumstances because it was a horrible exist-ence for me, but I didn't know what else to do with three kids in school. It was like being stuck in quicksand or mud."

**Andrea**: "I hung in there for my kids. They were my guiding light, my reason for living. I knew a lot from being a social worker, and alcoholism was not new to me from a profes-sional perspective. However, personally, it was new to me because there were not any alcoholics in my family. Mike was a hard worker who liked his beer. He socialized with a bunch of guys from work, and they all liked to drink beer. He was never nasty except when he had too much beer. That's when the kids and I would get on his nerves and off would come his leather belt. I had a supportive family, and they knew that Mike drank beer, but I don't think they ever knew that he hit us with his belt. But I could always go to my parents' house or my aunt's apartment nearby. Plus, I had numerous friends in town as well."

**Rosemary**: "After being married more than 50 years and having eight children together, you would think my husband would treat me better. He does this thing called 'gaslighting.' There was a movie about it many years ago where the husband tries to drive the wife crazy. My grown kids are my friends now besides being my kids. The entire family treats me as special. My women friends are a breath of fresh air, and we have so much fun together. At 80, I can be myself."

**Brenda**: "I tried to hide Jeff's bad behavior from my mother. I remember trying to save money, and Jeff was spending it left and right. I remember my mother sending us sets of sheets for the children's beds, and I took them to the store and returned them for cash. I can remember grocery shopping with my last $20. We would stay at my mother's house when we had to fly out of JFK airport. She was a smart woman and a good businesswoman, so she might have suspected the drinking and abuse from Jeff. I didn't want to burden her with knowing how things were."

**Brenda** continued, "My three kids were always supportive of me. Their dad often had an angry tone to his voice, and how could they ever forget seeing him passed out drunk on the floor in the morning? My kids and my work colleagues were there for me with understanding, support, and love."

**Elena**: "My family was very supportive. They were happy with my decision to divorce Warren. My mother believed I came to the right decision. She acknowledged that I tried to fulfill my promise to God but that Warren was making my life impossible. My relationships with family and friends were strengthened by the support they provided me. My sister has been nothing but an angel to me. She gave me the confidence I needed to change my life."

**Maureen**: "My family was glad that I didn't marry Paul. It was not a healthy relationship. He was intelligent and well-educated but was incredibly dishonest about his marital history and was very controlling. In the beginning, he treated me well, but it went downhill from there with every passing year. I invested four years in this relationship. No woman should have to live with abuse and many people believe that verbal abuse is what women tend to remember for the rest of their lives. It is as if they can hear the man's voice saying, 'You are stupid, you will never amount to anything without me, you are boring and one-dimensional, you are not capable of being on your own, and you are nothing.' Many of them can't get their abuser's voice out of their head."

**Beatrice**: "My strong family encouraged me to leave Bart. They were very supportive. I finally came home and lived in my parent's basement with my son. It was a new life for us. I did not want Billy to grow up with a father like Bart. I loved being around my family and friends again. I feel like I have Irish survival skills that helped me through this difficult situation with Bart. It might have been easier if I had not been so kind and giving. My family was supportive through my marriage, separation, and divorce. My close friends were there for me, too. I never felt abandoned by family or friends."

**Taryn**: "My parents had a wonderful, loving marriage, and I knew that Eli and I would be better off without Chuck. I grew to dislike him, not trust him, and realized that I made a mistake in marrying him. I felt trapped as his wife. His charm had worn off, and I did not like the Chuck I was seeing. He treated Eli okay, but he treated me terribly, especially with the punching and the verbal abuse. He was an unhappy person who lashed out at me every chance he could get. He blamed me for everything that didn't go well in his life. I think my parents tolerated Chuck, but I can't say that they had a close relationship. I think they sensed my unhappiness, my anxiety, my fear, and the stress I was under. Chuck was hard to please, difficult, mean, and always blamed others when things did not work out. I feared that the punching was only the beginning of a violent relationship. I knew I had to get out before things became worse."

**Susan**: "My family has always been supportive. I moved back to Pennsylvania with my daughters, Julie-Ann and Jody-Lynn. I am working part-time and have a nanny to help me with the girls. I love being a mother, and we see my parents and siblings weekly. It is great to have the girls grow up with grandparents and aunts, uncles, and cousins around. Scott has fulfilled his financial obligations, too."

**Barbara**: "I always had the support of my mother, brothers, sisters, and friends. Because Jay and I didn't have children, I didn't have that responsibility. I tried to put the memories of Jay's alcoholic behavior behind me and concentrate on the good things in my life. He could be so nasty, cruel, mean, and downright scary at times. He reduced me to tears many times. When he was under the influence, he could not control his temper. The best thing I could do was to get out of his way. My faith wavered during the last five years of our marriage when Jay was out of control with alcohol. I prayed that he would stop and change back to the man I married. That would have been a miracle."

**Marjorie**: "I had the support of my family, my college friends, and the other teachers from work. I never felt alone or without people who cared about me. However, Tad did a number on me over the years as I waited to start a family. When I think about it long and hard, I believe that Tad was enamored with his position in commercial real estate. He felt powerful, entitled, and on top of the world. He was a wheeler dealer. His world was a far cry from my world as a preschool teacher. Tad squashed my dreams to have a family. He had other goals in mind. I mourn what could have been but am delighted with the two darlings I adopted."

Women credited family and friends with being their lifeline or safety net. This suggests that they were indeed fortunate to have caring people in their lives. Conversely, this causes one to think about women who do not have a support system and hope that they have a "safe house" nearby in their community where they can seek refuge. A woman should move out of her domicile if the abuser is still residing there or has access to the dwelling. Restraining orders may not be the best protection for a woman who believes she is in a dangerous situation with a violent partner. Women suffering from abuse must be proactive in seeking an escape plan. They should also notify the appropriate authorities for police protection. It is helpful to inform a trusted friend or relative of problematic circumstances in a domestic relationship as well.

## Theme: Rediscovering Myself; Digging Deep

Some women said they lost themselves as a result of abuse. They talked about their journey to find themselves again. Women told how they went on to have a happy and meaningful life after they escaped abuse. Although every woman's circumstances were individual, they found possibilities and opportunities that brought them some measure of satisfaction. Some felt they had a new lease on life and were able to do things independently without fear. They told how they reflected on what was important in life. The following quotations illustrate their path.

**Sabrina**: "I remember telling my mother that wherever Kristin started kindergarten that's where we would stay because we had moved around enough. We celebrate April 5 every year because we just got back to the east coast in time for her to register for kindergarten. It was a big celebration for us for many years. Of course, Kristin is now 32. I was so ashamed of the chapter of my life with Antonio. I can't believe that I allowed someone to treat me so poorly, but I was a freshman in college and away from home for the first time. I am tough now; I am a probation officer. Now, I will not let anyone disrespect me, but I never get violent with anyone. I keep my cool pretty well. I think my daughter, Kristin, has anger built up in her about her father. I have encouraged her to have a civil relationship with him because he is her father. I can't do anything about it. I have told her to look at the positives in her relationship with him because he does have a good sense of humor. I say to her, 'If it hurts too much to have a relationship with him, then don't.' I tell her if you have expectations of him, he's never going to meet them. That's who he is and how he is. He has let her down so many times. I try to remind her how much her aunts, uncles, cousins, and grandparents love her. She is not lacking a loving family. We are both so fortunate to have them."

"After leaving Antonio, I grew as a person. My relationship with my family was therapeutic. My healing process was being with my family. I have such an appreciation for my family. We have such good times together. My parents have always been supportive of what their kids do. I am especially close to my sister, Eliza. Our bond is immeasurable. In our family, no one criticizes or scrutinizes, or questions anyone else to make them feel bad. We didn't grow up that way. When we are together, there are always a lot of laughs, and great food and everyone has a good time. There is just so much support, love, and acceptance. Throughout my life, I have always admired and appreciated my mother. I could easily see all that she did for our family. When I became a mother, I used my mother's example because she was a great role model. I am so blessed because my mother is truly a wonderful human being. I know that part of my unconditional love for Kristin is a result of the way my mother was to us."

**Sabrina** continued, "In my work, I deal with victims of domestic violence. I have a personal and professional understanding of what is going on. You are dealing with bad, negative stuff. I remember what it was like to be a victim. You have to take things seriously and be helpful. Because of my own experience with an abusive man, I see growth in the way I handle situations at work. I deal with people fairly and have compassion and empathy. Conversely, people know not to mess with me. If anyone ever puts their hands on me again, they would be sadly surprised (laughing)."

**Joanne**: "After June went away to college, I left Theo as I had planned to do. Of course, he was surprised and exploded in a fit of anger. He cursed, called me horrible names, and threw things in the house, breaking vases and other glassware. But I felt like an inmate let out of prison. I had walked on eggshells for so many years and found my newfound freedom exhilarating. I found the old Joanne again. It took a little while till I stopped looking over my shoulder. I still thrive on motherhood, and now June often travels with me to places I told her about when she was a little girl. I have rekindled my love of theater, art, and music. I took a French cooking class, joined a divorce support group at church, and have started to lead tours in France and Italy through a travel company. Life is finally good again."

**Marcella**: "I believe that I have had posttraumatic growth since I escaped Wyatt's abusive ways. I didn't want to be divorced, but he gave me no choice. I wanted to start a family, and he didn't. I could not live anymore with the control, his angry outbursts, the fear, the silent treatment, the stonewalling, the gaslighting, and his passive-aggressive behavior. He could have easily pushed me off the balcony in a fit of rage. I needed to get away from him. He was not the man I thought I married."

**Marcella** continued, "I got an apartment, credit cards, and a bank account. I felt free for the first time in 11 years. Yes, I still loved him, but I realized that I could not be with him unless he changed 99.9%, and that was not possible. I genuinely felt sorry for him. It took a little while to get used to living alone, but I enjoyed the peace and quiet. Every day was a new adventure. I kept the same job that I loved. I went to the beach with friends, to the movies, and out to dinner. I took a night class at a college with some co-workers. I went on my first cruise with a fellow group of teachers. I visited friends and family in Philadelphia, Chicago, and Atlanta. I could not do these things while married to Wyatt. He would not have allowed it."

**Bethany**: "I kept furthering my education after Jordan and I got divorced. I was able to do this with the support of family and friends. My three kids were wonderful to me. I had a *blast* with them when they were younger, and I still do today. We traveled to a lot of great places together. I know they love me and appreciate me. We have fun together. We all focus on the good times together and not the chaotic times with Jordan." Bethany added, "I have done well in my career, have great friendships, and a wonderful family. No woman should be a victim caught in a web of abuse. There are ways to get help, but you have to be careful because you don't want to end up as a homicide, especially when your kids need you."

**Andrea**: "After my husband died, I had a greater appreciation for life. I became more active in my church, went out to lunch with friends, and volunteered at the community hospital. I saw new possibilities, had a meaningful spiritual life, and felt the support of family and friends. I found the old Andrea again."

**Rosemary**: "Although I chose to stay married to Anthony, I was able to fill my life with my children and grandchildren. I also had my sewing circle, my women's group at church, my book club, the garden club, and a host of other activities. We had a very active parish, and I volunteered for many jobs at church. We also had a large extended family, so there were barbecues, parties, weddings, graduations, and baptisms. Life was never dull. All of these activities certainly acted as a buffer to Anthony's childish, mean, anger-ridden, and obnoxious behavior. My kids were well tuned in to his selfishness, cruelty, loud rants and raves, and generalized abuse."

**Brenda**: "I didn't let Jeff stifle my intellectual curiosity, and I continued my education. I made a nice life for myself without him. The kids all graduated from college and have a long-distance relationship with their father. I make it a point to not bad-mouth him to them. But I know that they have some memories of a chaotic household, with their father passed out on the floor. I'm sure they have some knowledge of his affairs and drinking and remember how badly he treated me. I don't share the terrible details with them. I am still working full-time at 79. I enjoy teaching college students. I have many friends and enjoy going to the theater, ballet, museums, and out to lovely restaurants in the Boston area. I also travel extensively during the summer months and have friends who live abroad. I visit them every summer."

**Elena**: "There is still a lot of damage from my marriage to Warren. I have a wonderfully supportive family, and they were happy with my decision to divorce Warren. Our marriage ended up being about abuse and power. I got so beaten down emotionally that I started to believe that I didn't deserve any better." Elena continued, "Fortunately, my family made me feel that I was in a safe place with them. They gave me the nurturance and love that I needed. I recognize that Warren has a mental illness. But I decided not to let him put me down anymore. I see myself in a positive light, and I am moving forward with an advanced degree. Sometimes there is a little sliver of self-doubt that creeps into my head as a result of the abuse, but I am getting better and better at overcoming it. My daughter, my parents, my brothers, and my sisters are my cheering section, and they readily pick me up if I am down. It happens less these days because I am engrossed in my courses and my job. I have come a long way, and I still have further to go, but I will get there."

**Maureen**: "As a result of my abusive relationship, I have plans for the future. I'd like to write a fictional book based on some of my experiences with men that might help young girls to recognize and steer clear of emotional abuse. Many females don't realize what it is: the controlling behaviors, the threats, the put-downs, the isolation, the fear, and the resulting shattered self-esteem. We need to get the word out because many people think abuse is only physical, and it's not. There is much more emotional abuse in the world than physical abuse. Women put up with it for a myriad of reasons, some of which may be financial, religious, cultural, status, and children. They don't want to 'rock the boat' so to speak. But in the meantime, life is chaotic, unstable, unhappy, and unhealthy. I am so glad that I didn't marry Paul after being in the relationship for four years."

**Beatrice**: "It took me a while to see growth in myself. However, it took strength to leave Bart. I didn't want my son, Billy, to grow up witnessing Bart's egregious behavior. After we left, I was a single parent for the first time. I could feel a scar forming in my heart. I wasn't a quitter, but I did this to save Billy and me from the throngs of abuse." Beatrice added, "Once we got away from Bart, I found my confidence returning. We were surrounded by family and friends and felt relaxed, relieved, and comfortable in my parents' finished basement. I am stronger than I thought I was. I think coming from a big family helps your sense of compassion. I was brought up to care about people and have empathy for those less fortunate or those befalling hard times."

**Taryn**: "I think I grew as a person once I left Chuck. Eli and I were better off living with my parents in a secure and loving home. I can't believe how relieved I feel. He made me feel small and insignificant as a person. When he started punching me, I felt paralyzed and did not know what to do. It was a new experience for me, and I froze most of the time. My siblings, friends, and co-workers have introduced me to a whole new life, a life of acceptance, enjoyment, and satisfaction. I have taken up golf and tennis. My mom and I go shopping together. I go to happy hour on Fridays after work with co-workers and friends. Mom and Dad take Eli out for pizza. Life is now full of new possibilities, and I love it."

**Susan**: "The best thing I ever did was leave Scott and move with my daughters back to Pennsylvania to be near my family. This change was better for all of us. I would not want to raise the girls with a detached, uninvolved, abusive father like Scott."

**Barbara**: "After Jay died, I continued with my life. It was a weight lifted off my shoulders. I missed the old Jay, but not the alcoholic Jay. His personality would change so much when he was under the influence. I used to say that vodka was his mistress. It was freeing not to worry about his temper and his total disregard for my family and friends. Now, I could have people over for dinner without fear of him acting out and embarrassing me.

There would be no more plates of spaghetti thrown at me, and no one would leave me at the airport waiting for three hours to be picked up. My new life is grand!"

**Marjorie**: "My growth stemmed from becoming a mother, finally. Adopting the children was the best decision I ever made. Although I was sad about the way things turned out with Tad, this was the best outcome for me. Having a caring, supportive network of family and friends made motherhood even better. My kids are loved by so many people now."

Women told how they went on to have a happy and meaningful life after they escaped abuse. Although every woman's circumstances were individual, they found possibilities and opportunities that brought them some measure of satisfaction. Some felt they had a new lease on life and were able to do things independently without fear. They told us how this process caused them to reflect on what was important in life. Sadly, not all abused women have support systems.

## Theme: Appreciating Life and Helping Others

Women in our study talked about their appreciation for life and their personal growth. They were proud of their strides forward and the peace and meaning that dwelled within them. Many expressed a strong desire to help others, especially those buried in the throes of abuse. The thankfulness they felt was a driving force to actively help others. The women believed they had a special insight into the abuse experience because it had been their lived experience. The following quotations exemplify the women's appreciation for life and their desire to help other abused women.

**Sabrina**: "My life is so much better now. It started to improve when Kristin and I returned to the east coast where my family lived. We did so much better surrounded by people who cared about us. I want to live my life helping others and making a difference. In my work, I help people. While domestic violence scars a woman for life, the scars heal even though a mark may be left on her soul, in her heart, and on her mind. With help, she can get out of a bad situation and end up in a better place."

**Joanne**: "My basic philosophy has stayed the same, and my daughter, June, is my priority in life. I am doing meaningful things for the rest of my life. I belong to a support group for separated and divorced women. I try to advocate for women who are in abusive relationships and help them learn from the experience. I want to help them see value in their life, see their potential, and new possibilities."

**Marcella**: "Before I married Wyatt, I saw myself as competent, caring, fun-loving, smart, and attractive. I have always been a 'people person.' When someone is in distress, I am the first person to come to their aid. That's just the way I am. I have always believed in treating others the way you want to be treated. I put God, family, and friends first in my life. I have helped several friends and relatives leave abusive relationships. Abuse crosses all ages, religions, races, socioeconomic groups, ethnicities, workforces, and cultures. We all should help others in need."

**Bethany**: "When Jordan and I got divorced, I remember the kids saying that they wanted to stay with me. I am still close with my three kids. I have also been a sounding board for other women who have had abusive partners. It is much more common than you might think. I believe that people are more aware of it today than when I was going through it years ago. I think that women are getting married older and with more life experience now. But abusive men are not always married men. Boyfriends can be abusive. Partners living together can be abusive. I think it is a societal problem, but I think women today are wiser and mothers are more apt to talk to their daughters about the possibility of being in an abusive relationship. There are also more safe houses in communities."

**Andrea**: "After Mike died, I had a greater appreciation for life. I became more active in my church and volunteered at the local hospital. I go out to lunch frequently with my women friends after I retired. My kids were always my priority. I have seven grandchildren. We all live within a 30-mile radius of each other. Sometimes I go on vacations with them, and other times I babysit. I have had more freedom since Mike passed away. In my past work as a social worker, I dealt with domestic abuse regularly. I have always had great empathy and compassion for others."

**Rosemary**: "Being the mother of eight children, I made sure that my daughters knew about domestic abuse and violence before they walked down the aisle and said 'I do.' They grew up seeing their father's anger, name-calling, yelling, and control. He was a very rigid man and a strict disciplinarian. I enjoy life much more now because I have learned to tune out Anthony when he is acting badly. Instead, I concentrate on having a good time with my kids, grandkids, and friends."

**Brenda**: "I have a great need to reach out to help others who are less fortunate, sick, and abused. I've grown to appreciate my life so much more after divorcing Jeff and moving on."

**Elena**: "I think I am probably an expert on emotional abuse. I have compassion for others, and I am not judgmental. All humans need to feel that they are in a safe place. For me, I have found my safe place, and I am thriving. I see so many possibilities in my future."

**Maureen**: "I am proud of myself for getting out of the relationship. I am glad that I did not marry Paul. I am a strong and capable woman. Life experiences have taught me a lot. I have learned many lessons, and I am still working on forgiving myself for some of the poor decisions I have made in my life. No woman should have to stay in an abusive relationship."

**Beatrice**: "I am stronger than I thought I was. I am a good mother to my son. I try to forgive myself for marrying Bart. My advice to women is to be cautious and not rush into anything. I'm now on a path to fulfilling myself as a person while helping others. You have to stand up for yourself and not let anyone crush your self-worth."

**Taryn**: "I am enjoying life having escaped Chuck's clutches. I feel the best when I am with Eli and when we are in my garden. Gardening allows me to enjoy nature. It was something I always liked but never had time for. I have taught Eli a lot about growing things. There is so much beauty in the world."

**Susan**: "I appreciate every day with my daughters and family. I have taught them how to ride horses like I did when I was their age. We have so much fun together. After having such a disappointing marriage, I find my life refreshing, and I am so thankful for this new beginning."

**Barbara**: "We need to educate the masses about abuse because it is all around us. Bad behavior should never be tolerated. I joined a support group after Jay died, which helped. Now, I volunteer at a women's shelter and lead a support group for abused women."

**Marjorie**: "I realize now that I could not have raised children with Tad. He was hardly ever home and was a workaholic. We grew apart, but I didn't realize it until the issue of starting a family came up. With kids, you want an equal partner and someone invested in parenthood and marriage. My decision to adopt was easy for me once Tad was out of my life. The kids and I have a very satisfying life. They complete me." Marjorie added, "I am in a support group for single mothers. Several of the other women came from abusive relationships. We help each other."

Women in this study told of their PTG that surfaced in varying degrees after they struggled with abuse. They recognized their credibility in helping other victims of abuse, having endured the experience. They embraced a mission to educate others about abuse as a global problem that crosses all socioeconomic groups, races, ethnicities, religions, education levels, and ages. They advocated for more safe houses in communities and greater police protection because restraining orders do not always guard against continued violence. It is of paramount importance that abused women get the social services and healthcare they need. In addition, abusers need anger management classes and specialized counseling in addition to incarceration as punishment for their violent behavior.

The themes that emerged from the interviews reinforced the findings from earlier studies (Anderson et al., 2012; D'Amore et al., 2018) of women who have suffered emotional and physical abuse by a spouse or partner. D'Amore and colleagues (2018) applied secondary qualitative analysis to an existing data set of ten verbatim transcripts of healing and post-traumatic growth (PTG). Findings revealed three overarching themes: (1) awareness and insight, (2) renewal and reconstruction, and (3) transformation and meaning. The current study's first theme, acknowledging the abusive relationship, is similar to D'Amore and colleagues' (2018) first overarching theme, awareness and insight, since both of these themes represent recognition of the abuse. D'Amore and colleagues' (2018) second theme, renewal and reconstruction, is comparable to theme four—rediscovering myself: digging deep—in the current study. D'Amore and colleagues' (2018) third theme, transformation and meaning, revealed that healing involved a multidimensional personal transformation

Table 6.1 Abused Women's Demographics

| Name | Number of Children | Marital Status | Age at Interview | Education Level | Current Occupation | Reported Socioeconomic Status |
|---|---|---|---|---|---|---|
| Beatrice | 1 | Divorced | 57 | Bachelors | Teacher | Middle |
| Joanne | 1 | Divorced | 64 | Associates | Real estate | Middle |
| Brenda | 3 | Divorced | 78 | Doctorate | Professor | Middle |
| Barbara | 0 | Widowed | 55 | Bachelors | Vet tech | Middle |
| Marcella | 0 | Divorced | 52 | Masters | Travel agent | Middle |
| Maureen | 3 | Separated | 62 | Masters | Teacher | Middle |
| Taryn | 1 | Divorced | 43 | Associate | Secretary | Middle |
| Rosemary | 8 | Married | 80 | High school | Homemaker | Middle |
| Andrea | 3 | Widowed | 74 | Masters | Social worker | Middle |
| Elena | 1 | Divorced | 51 | Masters | Graduate student | Middle |
| Marjorie | 2 | Divorced | 50 | Associate | Preschool aide | Middle |
| Susan | 2 | Divorced | 42 | Bachelors | Community worker | Middle |
| Sabrina | 1 | Unmarried | 51 | Bachelors | Probation officer | Middle |
| Bethany | 3 | Divorced | 60 | Masters | Technical writer | Middle |

within each woman combined with her supportive relationships. As in the current study, supportive relationships were a crucially important element in achieving a level of PTG.

In the current study, the investigators found storylines of the five-domain/five-factor model within their five identified themes. Women talked about their strength in making the difficult choice to end their marriage rather than succumb to a continuation of abuse, even though they foresaw an emotional impact on their children and a financial impact on the family. Some women embraced new possibilities as they changed career paths, returned to school or employment, joined support groups, connected with church-related activities, or embarked on new hobbies. Many women articulated a deepening of their spiritual or religious faith after they decided to end their abusive marriage. Most of these women told how they welcomed their freedom and a new or larger circle of friends after terminating their marriage. Many women stated that as time passed they felt a greater appreciation for life and a new sense of autonomy. They viewed themselves as strong, capable, and self-determined women but admitted their path was not easy, and it took time to incorporate many life changes.

In the current study, women's stories document the long-term scars of abuse and described fear, sadness, worry, and anxiety that resulted from cruelty, meanness, gaslighting, isolation, stonewalling, and other negative behaviors. In addition, arguing, berating, yelling, being slapped, hit, shoved, and being backed up to the wall were commonplace. One woman had a compound fracture of her wrist, and others had various bruises and abrasions. Severe blows to one's self-esteem, confidence, and abilities happened frequently. Not only were the women worried about their own emotional and physical well-being, but they were also concerned for their children.

Two women told of broken promises regarding having a baby. This caused shattered dreams that altered their futures. It also introduced feelings of betrayal, being lied to, and changing the game plan once "I do" was spoken. The element of control and power exerted by the abusers was described as overwhelming. The women described uncompromising situations which consisted of juggling an impossible workload, demanding sex, and blind obedience.

The findings of this study support the findings of Magne and colleagues (2021) and Arandia and colleagues (2016) that the five-factor or five-domain model of PTG (Tedeschi & Calhoun, 1996, 2004) was useful and comprehensive in illustrating PTG in study participants. The experiences described by participants suggest that nurses and other healthcare providers need to be vigilant in their assessment of abused women. Victims need to be informed of "safety nets" in their communities. Nurses need to adhere to the best practices as outlined in the current literature to help women seek safe alternatives to escape and break the cycle of abuse. Safety and privacy are also of paramount importance when nurses perform client assessments.

Narrative accounts from 14 women who had experienced emotional and/or physical abuse by their partner were obtained. These survivors described emotional and physical abuse in detail and wanted their voices to be heard. Families, friends, and co-workers made up the bulk of the women's support systems and played a significant role in each woman's decision to stay or leave the relationship. Women with children were especially concerned about the effect the abuse could have on their children. It was apparent from the women's stories that coping strategies were individual, and their awareness and actions were dynamic over time. None of the women mentioned calling the police or getting a restraining order. Except for one woman who was still married and had eight children, all relationships with abusive male partners were terminated. The findings of this study illustrate how rampant the problem of abuse is and reinforced the need for better, regular screening. Risk factors, such as a partner's abuse of alcohol, prescription, or illegal drugs, and/or a partner coming from an abusive home situation, may allow for more targeted interventions. However, further research is needed to identify specific assessment, intervention, and support strategies to end the cycle of intimate partner abuse.

Although there is a modest worldwide amount of both qualitative and quantitative research exploring PTG in women who have been abused by their partners, the majority of these studies occurred outside the Unted States where cultural and religious norms may differ significantly. The current study aimed to narrow and address this gap in US research.

## References

Anderzen-Carlsson, A., Gillå, C., Lind, M., Almqvist, K., Lindgren-Fändriks, A., & Källström, A. J. (2018, July 18). Child healthcare nurses' experiences of asking new mothers about intimate partner violence. *Journal of Clinical Nursing, 27*(7), 2752–2762. https://doi.org/10.1111/jocn.14242

Arandia, A. H., Mordeno, I. G., & Nalipay, M. N. (2016). Assessing the latent structure of posttraumatic growth and its relationship with cognitive processing of trauma among Filipino women victims of intimate partner abuse. *Journal of Interpersonal Violence, 33*(18), 2849–2866. http://doi.org/10.1177/0886260516632354

Benetato, B. B. (2011). Posttraumatic growth among operation enduring freedom and operation Iraqi freedom amputees. *Journal of Nursing Scholarship, 43*(4), 412–420. http://doi.org/10.1111/j.1547-5069.2011.01421.x

Black, M. C., Basile, K. C., Breiding, M. J., Smith, S. G., Walters, M. L., Merrick, M. T., & Stevens, M. R. (2011). *National intimate partner violence and sexual violence survey: 2010 summary report*. Centers for Disease Control and Prevention, National Center for Injury Prevention and Control.

Blevins, C. A., Weathers, F. W., Davis, M. T., Witte, T. K., & Domino, J. L. (2015). The posttraumatic stress disorder checklist for *DSM-5* (PCL-5): Development and initial psychometric evaluation. *Journal of Traumatic Stress, 28*(6), 489–498. https://doi.org/10.1002/jts.22059

Cleland, J. (2017). The qualitative orientation in medical education research. *Korean Journal of Medical Education, 29*(2), 61–71. https://doi.org/10.3946/kjme.2017.53

Cobb, A. R., Tedeschi, R. G., Calhoun, L. G., & Cann, A. (2006). Correlates of posttraumatic growth in survivors of intimate partner violence. *Journal of Traumatic Stress, 19*(6), 895–903. https://doi.org/10.1002/jts.20171

D'Amore, C., Martin, S. L., Wood, K., & Brooks, C. (2018). Themes of healing and posttraumatic growth in women survivors' narratives of intimate partner violence. *Journal of Interpersonal Violence, 36*(5–6), NP2697–NP2724. https://doi.org/10.1177/0886260518767909

Doyle, K. M., Knetig, J. A., & Iverson, K. W. (2022). Practical implications of research on intimate partner violence experiences for the mental health clinician. *Current Treatment Options in Psychiatry, 9*, 280–300. https://doi.org/10.1007/s40501-022-00270-6

Dyjakon, D., & Rajba, B. (2021). Post-traumatic growth: Longitudinal study on battered women in close relationships after both they and their partners undergo therapy. *Journal of Interpersonal Violence*, 088626052199793. https://doi.org/10.1177/0886260521997932

Farnia, V., Tatari, F., Salemi, S., Alikhani, M., & Basanj, B. (2017). Efficacy of trauma-focused cognitive behavioral therapy in facilitating posttraumatic growth and emotional management among physically abused children. *Trauma Monthly, 23*(2). https://doi.org/10.5812/traumamon.62149

Gerber, M. R., Fried, L. E., Pineles, S. L., Shipherd, J. C., & Bernstein, C. A. (2012). Posttraumatic stress disorder and intimate partner violence in a women's headache center. *Women and Health, 52*(5), 454–471. https://doi.org/10.1080/03630242.2012.684088

Gonzalez-Mendez, R., & Hamby, S. (2020). Identifying women's strengths for promoting resilience after experiencing intimate partner violence. *Violence and Victims, 36*(1), 29–44. https://doi.org/0.1891/vv-d-18-00178

Hays, D. G., & Singh, A. A. (2011). *Qualitative inquiry in clinical and educational settings* (1st ed.). The Guilford Press.

Holgersen, K., Boe, H., & Holen, A. (2010). Long-term perspectives on posttraumatic growth in disaster survivors. *Journal of Traumatic Stress,* https://doi.org/10.1002/jts.20530

Larick, J., & Graf, N. M. (2012). Battlefield compassion and posttraumatic growth in combat servicepersons. *Journal of Social Work in Disability & Rehabilitation, 11*(4), 219–239. http://doi.org/1 0.1080/1536710x.2012.730824

Lincoln, Y. S., & Guba, E. (1985). *Naturalistic inquiry* (1st ed.). SAGE Publications.

Magne, H., Delbreil, A., Gambier, M., Goutaudier, N., Jaafari, N., & Voyer, M. (2021). La croissance post-traumatique chez les victimes de violences conjugales: Une étude pilote dans la vienne. *L'Encéphale.* https://doi.org/10.1016/j.encep.2021.04.001

Mark, K. M., Stevelink, S. M., Choi, J., & Fear, N. T. (2018). Post-traumatic growth in the military: A systematic review. *Occupational and Environmental Medicine, 75*(12), 904–915. https://doi.org/10.1136/oemed-2018-105166

Martin, L., Byrnes, M., Bulsara, M. K., McGarry, S., Rea, S., & Wood, F. (2017). Quality of life and posttraumatic growth after adult burn: A prospective, longitudinal study. *Burns, 43*(7), 1400–1410. https://doi.org/10.1016/j.burns.2017.06.004

Moschella, E. A., Turner, S., & Banyard, V. L. (2018). Posttraumatic growth as a mediator of self-blame and happiness in the context of interpersonal violence. *Violence and Victims, 33*(6), 1088–1101.

Oh, J., Kim, Y., & Kwak, Y. (2021). Factors influencing posttraumatic growth in ovarian cancer survivors. *Supportive Care in Cancer, 29*(4), 2037–2045. https://doi.org/10.1007/s00520-020-05704-6

Palmer, E., Murphy, D., & Spencer-Harper, L. (2016). Experience of post-traumatic growth in UK veterans with PTSD: A qualitative study. *Journal of the Royal Army Medical Corps, 163*(3), 171–176. https://doi.org/10.1136/jramc-2015-000607

Rivara, F. P., Anderson, M. L., Fishman, P., Bonomi, A. E., Reid, R. J., Carrell, D., & Thompson, R. S. (2007). Healthcare utilization and costs for women with a history of intimate partner violence, *American Journal of Preventive Medicine, 32*(2), 89–96. https://doi.org/10.1016/j.amepre.2006.10.001

Royse, D., & Badger, K. (2018). Burn survivors' near-death experiences: A qualitative examination. *OMEGA—Journal of Death and Dying, 80*(3), 440–457. https://doi.org/10.1177/0030222818755286

Sandelowski, M. (2009). What's in a name? Qualitative description revisited. *Research in Nursing & Health, 33*(1), 77–84. https://doi.org/10.1002/nur.20362

Sawyer, A., Ayers, S., Young, D., Bradley, R., & Smith, H. (2012). Posttraumatic growth after childbirth: A prospective study. *Psychology & Health, 27*(3), 362–377. https://doi.org/10.1080/08870446.2011.578745

Soo, H., & Sherman, K. A. (2014). Rumination, psychological distress, and post-traumatic growth in women diagnosed with breast cancer. *Psycho-Oncology, 24*(1), 70–79. https://doi.org/10.1002/pon.3596

Tedeschi, R. G., & Calhoun, L. G. (1996). The posttraumatic growth inventory: Measuring the positive legacy of trauma. *Journal of Traumatic Stress, 9*(3), 455–471. https://doi.org/10.1002/jts.2490090305

Tedeschi, R. G., & Calhoun, L. G. (2004). Target article: "Posttraumatic growth: Conceptual foundations and empirical evidence". *Psychological Inquiry, 15*(1), 1–18. https://doi.org/10.1207/s15327965pli1501_01

Tsai, J., Sippel, L. M., Mota, N., Southwick, S. M., & Pietrzak, R. H. (2015). Longitudinal course of posttraumatic growth among U.S. military veterans: Results from the national health and resilience in veterans study. *Depression and Anxiety, 33*(1), 9–18. https://doi.org/10.1002/da.22371

Weiss, D. S., & Marmar, C. R. (1996). The impact of event scale—Revised. In J. Wilson & T. M. Keane (Eds.), *Assessing psychological trauma and PTSD* (pp. 399–411). Guilford.

# 7

# THERAPEUTIC MODALITIES, SELF-HELP RESOURCES, AND IMPLICATIONS FOR CLINICAL PRACTICE, EDUCATION, AND RESEARCH

Since PTSD was first listed in the *Diagnostic and Statistical Manual of Mental Disorders* in 1980, mental healthcare providers have identified several therapies that may be effective in helping people cope with traumatic memories. Mindfulness training, cognitive behavioral therapy (CBT), and eye movement desensitization and reprocessing therapy (EMDR) are three of these therapeutic modalities that are especially suitable for people suffering from PTSD.

## Therapeutic Modalities: Mindfulness Training

Mindfulness is the capacity to intentionally bring awareness to present-moment experiences with an attitude of acceptance, openness, and honesty (Kabat-Zinn, 1996, 2001, 2006, 2009). It is being awake to the fullness of life at that immediate time. It is appreciated by the five senses and is a meditative practice that can soothe a distracted or distressed mind and increase one's sense of feeling grounded.

Mindfulness training can reduce emotional, psychological, and physiological stress. It is different from simply trying to relax, and it does not involve stopping one's thinking. Mindfulness has been known to improve empathy, compassion, appreciation for life, self-concept, and overall sense of wellness. Many people who practice mindfulness regularly report feeling calm, peaceful, reflective, fulfilled, and relaxed. In addition, many believe that it dispels the feeling of "being on automatic pilot" or pacing on a constant treadmill. It can quiet the mind and decrease negative self-talk, pessimistic thinking, and obsessive worrying. Mindfulness training involves a conscious effort to shift the mind to present-moment experience, moving away from counterproductive thinking patterns that interfere with well-being.

Neuroscience research has indicated that mindfulness practices enhance brain function in the areas of critical thinking and problem-solving. At the same time, they can modulate emotions such as fear, anger, and anxiety. This type of training can strengthen one's ability to assess situations with acute attention and a clearer focus. Mindfulness practices have relevance for all humans and can be traced to the seminal work of Jon Kabat-Zinn in 1979.

DOI: 10.4324/9781003456650-7

His mindfulness-based stress reduction program (MBSR) was developed originally to reduce chronic pain in patients. It was a structured eight-week program that incorporated a variety of stress reduction exercises and techniques geared to increase one's capacity to become more mindful. Core practices included gentle yoga, breathing awareness, and tuning in to bodily sensations. For patients with chronic pain, research examining the effects of Kabat-Zinn's MBSR program mentioned improvements in these patients.

As a result of the success of the MBSR program, there was noteworthy media attention and mindfulness training programs began throughout the United States. These programs did not just stay in the clinical arena but spread to the corporate sector, and became popular with athletes, educators, and performers. Mindfulness can interrupt the cycle of overwhelming thoughts and feelings that plague many humans. It can also enhance communication with family, friends, and co-workers. It is a lifelong process that can be that "life preserver" in times of trauma and stress.

Suggestions for the practice of mindfulness in daily life include the following steps:

1. For 5–10 minutes a day, sit in a comfortable chair and focus on your breathing; tune in to it.
2. When your mind wanders, bring it back to your awareness by concentrating on your breathing.
3. Awareness of your breathing is a form of meditation and helps to slow your mental activity.
4. Focus on your bodily sensations. This will quiet your distracted mind.
5. Gentle stretching or slow walking can also quiet your busy mind.
6. Notice your activities of daily living with greater awareness. Explore them using your five senses.

*(Kabat-Zinn, 1996, 2001, 2006, 2009)*

## Therapeutic Modalities: Cognitive Behavioral Therapy

Cognitive behavioral therapy (CBT) is a type of psychotherapy in which negative patterns of thinking about oneself and the world are challenged to alter unwanted behaviors or treat mood disorders such as depression and anxiety. With CBT, people learn to recognize distortions in their thinking that are causing problems for them in life. Then, they reevaluate this thinking considering reality. They gain a better understanding of the behaviors and motivations of others. CBT focuses on learning to change thoughts (cognitions) and behaviors (actions). It breaks things down that cause a person to feel bad about themselves or sad or anxious or frightened. It helps to make a person's problems more manageable and can assist in changing negative thought patterns and improving the way they feel.

Aaron Beck is known as the "Father of CBT" and defined three levels of cognition: core beliefs, dysfunctional assumptions, and automatic negative thoughts. He outlined five steps to change one's thinking: (1) make a list of thinking errors, (2) record unproductive thoughts, (3) create replacement thoughts, (4) read your list often, and (5) notice and reframe thoughts (Beck et al., 2003).

It is important to recognize that a person's core beliefs are learned and influenced by early childhood experiences. They are deeply rooted in one's belief system and identify negative views held about oneself, the world, and the future. Similarly, dysfunctional assumptions are cognitive distortions that occur because of a natural proclivity to focus on the negative. This causes an inaccurate, distorted perception of reality and a general misinterpretation of information. These cognitive distortions are irrational thought patterns that capitalize on negativity. Examples of these distortions are polarized thinking, negative mental filtering, overgeneralization, jumping to conclusions, catastrophizing, personalization, blaming, labeling, always being right, making "should" statements, emotional reasoning, control fallacies, the fallacy of change, the fallacy of fairness, and the heaven's reward fallacy (Beck, 1975, 1999; Beck et al., 1979; Beck et al., 1989; Beck et al., 2003; Beck et al., 2005; Beck et al., 2008; Beck & Alfred, 1998; Beck & Clark, 2010).

Beck's contributions to psychiatry spanned from the 1960s till his death in 2021. His greatest contribution was the Beck Depression Inventory and his extensive publications on CBT which spanned more than 60 years. He used CBT with a wide variety of patients, including those with anxiety, depression, personality disorders, suicidal ideation, and even schizophrenia. CBT is the most widely used form of psychotherapy in the world.

### Therapeutic Modalities: Eye Movement Desensitization and Reprocessing Therapy

Eye movement desensitization and reprocessing therapy (EMDR) has inched its way into mainstream therapy. The practice involves having a client process a traumatic memory while simultaneously interacting with images, sounds, and sensations that activate both sides of the brain. The objective is to anchor the brain in the present moment as the client recalls the past.

In recent years, EMDR has helped scores of military veterans from the wars in Iraq and Afghanistan diminish, reduce, or abandon their PTSD symptoms. This therapy has been touted by Bessel van der Kolk in his seminal book *The Body Keeps the Score* as one of the most effective ways to treat PTSD. The efficacy of EMDR therapy has been well-established in the last two decades with research with over 30 randomized controlled studies with positive results.

EMDR was discovered by Francine Shapiro, a psychologist in 1987. She noticed that moving her eyes from side to side while contemplating difficult thoughts or memories improved her mood. She has suggested that the average person has between 10 and 20 unprocessed memories responsible for most of the pain and trauma in their life. In 2013, the World Health Organization reported that trauma-focused cognitive behavioral therapy (TF-CBT) and EMDR are the only psychotherapeutic modalities recommended for the treatment of PTSD.

EMDR aims to cause the person to put to rest old feelings related to trauma and learn new ways of responding and interpreting thoughts and feeling differently. In other words, the way a person thinks, feels, and responds to memories of the event can be rewritten and healing can become possible.

EMDR works in eight phases: history taking, client preparation, assessment, desensitization, installation, body scan, closure, and reevaluation of the treatment effect. Clients are reminded that healing is a journey and to take it one day at a time. There will be good days and bad days. EMDR can unburden a person of past trauma and help them heal as they access their innate wisdom (Shapiro, 1989a, 1989b, 1991, 1995, 2001; Shapiro & Forrest, 1997).

### Self-Help Initiatives

Most people are not aware that there are almost four times as many widows as widowers in the United States, and over 700,000 women become widows every year. However, in many communities, there are very few resources out there for widows beyond conventional grief counseling. But, when they lose their life partners, widows also lose their financial partner, their social partner, their emotional partner, and many of their hopes for the future. Dreams of what could have been in their life path as a couple are terminated.

Besides the aforementioned therapies, many people who experience loss or trauma in their lives turn to self-help strategies to cope with the sadness and stress of loss as a means to help them go on. There is a moderate number of online websites, online meeting forums, in-person meetings, and telephone helplines to assist people who are grieving the loss of a spouse or child, as well as other traumas such as a cancer diagnosis, emotional and physical intimate partner abuse, or rape.

### Widows' Self-Help

A modest number of churches, funeral parlors, synagogues, and faith-based organizations hold in-person support group meetings for widows. Frequently, these venues advertise group meeting schedules in their church bulletin or organizational brochures. Additionally, a pastor or funeral director may discuss their offerings to the newly widowed. Some widows are more comfortable with in-person contact with others who have had a similar loss. Others may seek out online connectivity with widows' groups and find comfort and flexibility with this type of support venue.

Several online widows support groups have a wide presence on the Internet. These are the Modern Widows Club (https://modernwidowsclub.com), the Widows' Connection (Widows' Connection: https://widowsconnection.org), and Soaring Spirits (https://soaringspirits.org). All three groups believe in widows helping widows. The Modern Widows Club was founded in 2011. It is a women's health organization serving widows seeking to understand their experience and focus on growth. Their research into widows' physical and mental health informs their programs and encourages awareness for women who have been historically invisible, unsupported, uncounted, and "under the radar" in many communities (https://modernwidowsclub.com).

The Modern Widows Club offers in-person and virtual support groups, clubs and activities, educational courses, mentoring programs, conferences, videos, podcasts, and opportunities for advocacy. They support widows of all ages, ethnic backgrounds, beliefs, faiths, and loss circumstances, and serve to empower widows to "lean into life, build resilience and make a positive difference in society" (https://modernwidowsclub.com).

The Widows' Connection is a national nonprofit organization of widows helping widows rebuild their lives after the life-changing event of losing a spouse. According to their website, the Widows' Connection has helped close to 10,000 widows find new meaning and fulfillment again in their lives. The Widow's Connection espouses filling a crucial gap in a widow's recovery offering education, connection, encouragement, and empowerment through original programming, research, and the healing power of social connection. This organization offers weekly peer-led meetings and monthly webinars, virtual meetings, and podcasts based on where a woman is on her widow journey. Widows' Connection also offers monthly virtual wellness webinars and workshops hosted by experts in their field and in-person quarterly conferences around the United States (https://widowsconnection.org).

Soaring Spirits is an international organization that has one goal: to connect widowed people with each other. Soaring Spirits provides information, resources, and understanding for those who are newly widowed. Membership includes men and women. This organization offers several diverse programs, such as Camp Widow, an in-person, uplifting, life-affirming event planned for widowed people by widowed people; regional social group meetings for widowed people all over the United States and internationally; and Widowed Village, a 24/7 online community for persons to write, read, and share thoughts with other widowed people. This organization is nonprofit but does charge monthly dues. However, it does offer initial services and resources to the newly widowed without having to become a dues-paying member (http://soaringspirits.org).

### Loss of a Child Self-Help

Several national organizations are devoted to helping grieving parents who have lost a child. The Compassionate Friends organization exists to provide friendship, understanding, and hope to parents going through the natural grieving process whether their child died at any age and from any cause. Compassionate Friends offers "virtual chapters" through an online support community that includes live chats. This program was established to encourage connecting and sharing among parents, grandparents, and siblings (over the age of 18) grieving the death of a child. The chat rooms supply support, encouragement, and friendship. The friendly atmosphere encourages conversation among friends who understand the emotions they are experiencing. There are general bereavement sessions as well as more specific sessions. Compassionate Friends also offers a variety of private Facebook groups. These pages are moderated by bereaved parents, siblings, or grandparents and may not be accessed unless a request to join is approved by a moderator. Interested parties should access Compassionate Friends information on their webpage (www.compassionatefriends.org).

Bereaved Parents of the USA was founded in 1995 in Illinois. Bereaved Parents of the USA is a national organization aimed at providing a safe space where grieving families can connect, share their stories, and learn to rebuild their lives. This organization offers meetings whenever they can where parents can share their fears, confusion, anger, guilt, frustrations, emptiness, and feelings of hopelessness, knowing these emotions will be met with compassion and understanding. This organization espouses support, comfort, and encouragement toward one another and offers hope and healing. They believe that as members confront the deaths of their loved ones, their shared grief brings them to a common ground that transcends differences, building mutual understanding across the boundaries of culture, race, faith, values, abilities, and lifestyle (https://bereavedparentsusa.org). There are over 25 chapters of Bereaved Parents of the USA, and more information can be found on their website, https://bereavedparentsusa.org

### Self-Help for Survivors of a Close Brush With Death

Theravive is a network of licensed and professional clinical counselors, therapists, and psychologists who strive to make mental health care safe, affordable, and accessible. Their goal is to help people reach their potential, overcome difficult journeys, and effect real and lasting change. They maintain strong academic rigor; as therapists they hold advanced degrees and are required to be fully licensed to practice counseling. Their purpose is to connect people to the right professional, giving them a better direction, attainable goals, and a clearer understanding of how to get there. Their therapists specialize in every form of counseling, including relationships, anxiety, trauma/PTSD, depression, families, career change, loss, addictions, children, eating disorders, couples, marriages, and intimate partner abuse. This organization can connect people to online and in-person counseling services by an individual's zip code. These professionals can be a valuable resource for anyone struggling with life challenges such as a close brush with death experience, widowhood, the loss of a child, or intimate partner abuse (www.theravive.com). Their website is http://www.theravive.com.

### Survivors of Intimate Partner Abuse Self-Help

Intimate partner violence includes physical, sexual, or emotional abuse, as well as sexual coercion and stalking by a current or former intimate partner. An intimate partner is a person with whom one has or has had a close personal or sexual relationship. Intimate partner violence affects millions of women each year in the United States. Intimate partner abuse can alter an individual's view of the world and affect how one approaches life. These experiences can also directly affect the individual's personal or professional life for many years. Just as each person is unique, so is the journey toward recovery for each individual. However, it is possible for survivors to heal and live a fulfilling life. Recovery does not have to be pursued alone. Sharing with other survivors in a group setting can reduce the sense of isolation that is often felt after experiencing a life-altering event. Connecting with others can also provide a safe environment where trust and other crucial life skills can gradually be restored.

The US Department of Health and Human Services, Office of Women's Health (www.womenshealth.gov) website provides a wealth of information on intimate partner abuse including a listing of services provided by each state as well as checklists of abusive behaviors and emergency contact information. State listings of resources include those offered for women and those offered for women with children (www.womenshealth.gov).

### Implications for Nursing Clinical Practice

Nurses who care for women who have lost a spouse or longtime partner can acquaint them with the possibility of PTG and all that it entails in terms of the various domains: greater appreciation of life, improved relationships with others, personal strength, openness to new possibilities, and spiritual growth. Women who experienced this kind of loss often have difficulty navigating life without their significant other. Nurses are in pivotal positions to educate them about the grieving process and the possibility of PTG. They can help women find their way through trauma and teach them about healing, coping, empathy, compassion, and the power of being connected to others. Nurses can advocate for these women and introduce widows to self-help initiatives on a national and community level.

Nurses who care for women who have lost a child to death acknowledge the magnitude of the loss because it goes against the natural course of life, in that parents are not expected to outlive their children. Many researchers have reported that grief and sorrow from losing a child tend to be more intense, disruptive, and longer-lasting than other types of losses, particularly for mothers. These women grieve their loss in a variety of ways based on culture, personality, spirituality, core beliefs, and a mix of individual attributes. Nurses and other healthcare providers need to understand factors that help mothers cope effectively to prevent maladaptive behaviors and promote PTG. Grief following loss is individual and cannot have a "one size fits all" approach or a uniformly measured trajectory. Nurses can serve as advocates for bereaved parents and acquaint them with national and local resources.

Nurses are in key positions to foster awareness of the possibility of PTG and provide some hope to women struggling after a close brush with death. This type of trauma may come as a shock in some situations such as a catastrophic accident or a man-made or natural disaster. Conversely, it may be the exacerbation of a chronic health problem or a sudden serious illness. Nurses can educate women about PTG and the fact that it takes time to develop. They need to engage in therapeutic listening and comfort trauma survivors. They can also make appropriate referrals to facilitate timely care.

Nurses are often the first healthcare providers abused women encounter when seeking help. Settings may include emergency rooms, clinics, primary care offices, and community health centers. The nurse–client relationship is significant to clinical nursing practice to provide quality care. Nurses must be prepared to build a therapeutic alliance and address the needs of abused women. Women need to be screened for abuse at annual and episodic healthcare visits to make sure they are safe in their homes. Questions about safety at home and in relationships need to be included in assessment tools. The US Preventive Services Task Force (Curry et al., 2018) has endorsed several assessment tools that have demonstrated excellent sensitivity and specificity from the research literature. These tools are available on the Internet for the public and clinicians to download. They can be used in any healthcare setting and even as a self-assessment tool by anyone.

Nurses know that the cycle of abuse does not always manifest in physical injuries. There is usually a strong emotional component in domestic abuse. Women who endure emotional abuse may be "invisible" victims and may be overlooked by the healthcare system. However, nurses educated to care for these women know what to look for and will try to keep them safe and from falling through the cracks. Nurses can be strong advocates for abused women and ensure these women learn about national, state, and local resources that are available to help.

Regardless of the type of trauma or loss, nurses and other healthcare providers need to be aware of the possibility of PTG in the four aforementioned groups of women as well as in other vulnerable populations. PTG can coexist with distress caused by trauma and loss. When PTG occurs, it exceeds resilience because it results in a higher level of functioning. PTG takes time to develop and occurs in varying degrees. It may be a greater appreciation of life, increased personal strength, openness to new possibilities, improved relationships, enhanced compassion, and spiritual growth. There is no specific timeline for PTG, and there is no guarantee that a person will experience it.

### Implications for Nursing Education

Teaching about trauma, PTSD, and its symptomatology, as well as the concept of posttraumatic growth should begin at the undergraduate level. More information about widowhood, loss of a child, a close brush with death, and intimate partner abuse needs to be added across the undergraduate and graduate curriculums, especially with familiarity with assessment tools, open-ended interviewing techniques, core questions, and current information on available self-help strategies and professional therapy resources. Students need to learn approaches to traumatized people that are grounded in clinical research and have a solid track record of success in clinical practice. At the graduate and doctoral levels, nurses need to gain knowledge of current research and research-supported interventions in caring for widows, parents who have lost a child to death, people who have had a traumatic close brush with death, and women who have suffered from intimate partner abuse. These four aforementioned traumas occur in many women at some point in their lives, and informed and skilled nurses are a vital force in helping these women navigate the trauma in their lives.

## Implications for Nursing Research

There are many potential areas for nursing research exploration surrounding widowhood, loss of a child, a close brush with death experience, and women who have experienced intimate partner abuse. A one-size-fits-all approach in assessing these women in a variety of clinical settings or their homes is not a solid strategy. Care needs to be tailored to the woman and her unique circumstances. Clinical nursing judgment, critical thinking, and timing of an encounter play a crucial role in assessing these clients and providing interventions. For example, the research literature about intimate partner abuse (Anderzen-Carlsson et al., 2018; Jack et al., 2017; Sundberg et al., 2017) demonstrates that a tailored approach to each woman and her environmental circumstances is needed. For some women, violence in family relationships is a normative legacy; often their mothers, aunts, and sisters were abused. These women were exposed to violence in multiple family settings and their communities (Jack et al., 2017). Some researchers advocate for the use of research-supported assessment tools at the time of client intake interviews (Curry et al., 2018), whereas others (Jack et al., 2017) believe that the employment of screening tools too early does not promote disclosure of abuse. Nurses need to use their clinical judgment and critical thinking skills to evaluate client encounters and decide on the timing and approach to discussing the possibility of abuse. The same is true for many other types of trauma assessment and intervention.

In terms of widowhood, loss of a child, a close brush with death, and intimate partner abuse, many of these topics lend themselves to qualitative or mixed-method studies, whereas other studies using quantitative measures would be more appropriate. A methodological direction would depend on the research question being investigated. Longitudinal studies should be encouraged because alterations in a woman's circumstances change over time such as her support systems, safety, resources, and her willingness and ability to disclose her feelings and thoughts.

## References

Anderzen-Carlsson, A., Gillå, C., Lind, M., Almqvist, K., Lindgren-Fändriks, A., & Källström, A.J. (2018, July 18). Child healthcare nurses' experiences of asking new mothers about intimate partner violence. *Journal of Clinical Nursing, 27*(7), 2752–2762. https://doi.org/10.1111/jocn.14242

Beck, A. (1975). *Cognitive therapy and emotional disorders*. Plume/Penguin.

Beck, A. (1999). *Prisoners of hate: The cognitive basis of anger, hostility, and violence*. Harper Perennial.

Beck, A., & Alfred, B. (1998). *The integrative power of cognitive therapy*. Guilford.

Beck, A., & Clark, D. (2010). *Cognitive therapy of anxiety disorders: Science and practice*. Guilford.

Beck, A., Emery, G., & Greenberg, R. (2005). *Anxiety disorders and phobias: A cognitive perspective*. Basic Books.

Beck, A., Rector, N., Stolar, N., & Grant, P. (2008). *Schizophrenia: Cognitive theory, research, and therapy*. Google Books.

Beck, A., Rush, J., Shaw, B., & Emery, G. (1979). *Cognitive therapy of depression*. Guilford.

Beck, A., Scott, J., & Williams, M. (1989). *Cognitive therapy in clinical practice: An illustrative casebook*. Imprint Routledge.

Beck, A., Winterowd, C., & Gruener, D. (2003). *Cognitive therapy with chronic pain patients*. Springer Publishing Company.

Bereaved Parents of the USA. (n.d.). https://bereavedparentsusa.org

Curry, S. J., Krist, A. H., Owens, D. K., Barry, M. J., Caughey, A. B., Davidson, K. W., Doubeni, C. A., Epling, J. W., Grossman, D. C., Kemper, A. R., Kubik, M., Kurth, A., Landefeld, C. S., Mangione, C. M., Silverstein, M., Simon, M. A., Tseng, C. W., & Wong, J. B. (2018). Screening for intimate partner violence, elder abuse, and abuse of vulnerable adults: U.S. Preventive Services Task Force Final Recommendation Statement. *Journal of the American Medical Association, 320*(16), 1678–1687. https://doi.org/10.1001/jama.2018.1474

Jack, S. M., Ford-Gilboe, M., Davidson, D., & MacMillan, H. L. (2017). Identification andassessment of intimate partner violence in nurse home visitation. *Journal of Clinical Nursing, 26*(15), 2215–2228. https://doi.org/10.1111/jocn.13392

Kabat-Zinn, J. (1996*). Full catastrophe living: How to cope with stress, pain, and illness with mindfulness meditation*. Piatkus Books.

Kabat-Zinn, J. (2001). *Mindfulness meditation for everyday life*. Piatkus Books.

Kabat-Zinn, J. (2006). *Coming to our senses: and the world through mindfulness meditation*. Hyperion Books.

Kabat-Zinn, J. (2009). *Letting everything become your teacher: Lessons in mindfulness*. Dell Publishing.

Modern Widows Club. (n.d.). https://modernwidowsclub.com

Shapiro, F. (1989a). Efficacy of the eye movement desensitization procedure in the treatment of traumatic memories. *Journal of Traumatic Stress, 2*, 199–223.

Shapiro, F. (1989b). Eye movement desensitization: A new treatment for post-traumatic stress disorder. *Journal of Behavior Therapy and Experimental Psychiatry, 20*, 211–217.

Shapiro, F. (1991). Eye movement desensitization & reprocessing procedure: From EMD to EMD/R—a new treatment model for anxiety and related traumata. *Behavioral Therapist, 14*, 133–135.

Shapiro, F. (1995). *Eye movement desensitization and reprocessing: Basic principles, protocols, and procedures* (1st ed.). Guilford Press.

Shapiro, F. (2001). *Eye movement desensitization and reprocessing: Basic principles, protocols, and procedures* (2nd ed.). Guilford Press.

Shapiro, F., & Forrest, M. (1997). *EMDR: The breakthrough therapy for overcoming anxiety, stress, and trauma*. Basic Books.

Soaring Spirits. (n.d.). https://soaringspirits.org

Sundberg, E., Törnkvist, L., Saleh-Stattin, N., Wändell, P., & Hylander, I. (2017). To ask, or not to ask: The hesitation process described by district nurses encountering women exposed to intimate partner violence. *Journal of Clinical Nursing, 26*(8), 2256–2265. https://doi.org/10.1111/jocn.12992

The Compassionate Friends. (n.d.). https://compassionate.friends.org

The Widow's Connection. (n.d.). https://widowsconnection.org

Theravive. (n.d.). https://www.theravive.com

U.S. Department of Health and Human Services, Office of Women's Health. (n.d.). https://www.womenshealth.gov

# 8

# AUTHORS' CONCLUDING THOUGHTS

Women's experiences of PTG, as well as PTSD, need to be a priority in future research. Currently, there are many more studies involving PTSD rather than PTG. In fact, as nurse researchers, we only discovered the concept of PTG through our previous work with PTSD in military nurses deployed to Iraq and Afghanistan. Yet, we did encounter some experiences of PTG in the military nurses we interviewed about deployment and reintegration experiences.

Just as the women we interviewed about their trauma will never forget their experiences, they will also never forget their challenging journey to PTG. They were cognizant of the fact that there was no guarantee that they would come to recognize PTG in themselves.

In data collection and analysis, we noticed that the women who volunteered for our various studies investigating PTG all had some degree of PTG. This caused us to pause and wonder if most women who agree to participate in a research study of this nature do so because they want to tell their stories to help other women who are struggling in the aftermath of trauma. Is it because of their growth in some of the five domains outlined by Tedeschi and Calhoun that they want to come forward with their narrative? Perhaps someone who has not experienced any growth after trauma is not inclined to share their experience with others. They may not have anything positive to say or may even be clinically depressed. They may not feel up to discussing their experience and may not see value in participating in a study which could cause them to relive the trauma, which could lead to negative or stressful feelings or thoughts. In addition, because our research is qualitative and involves interviews, it seems likely that the participants may gain something from telling their stories and elaborating on how they managed to go on with life after their trauma. Participation could have been cathartic for them. A sense of altruism could have fostered their interest in participating in a study about loss and/or trauma.

While we don't have the answers to the aforementioned questions, responses from many of the participants display a sense of or a belief in PTG. Consequently, this sense or belief may move a person to be involved in a research endeavor of this nature. Initially, it surprised us that all of the women who agreed to participate in this research had at least

DOI: 10.4324/9781003456650-8

some recognition of PTG in their lives. However, after giving much thought to the PTG conceptual model, we were less surprised and more accepting of the motivation of participants. Also, in a therapeutic alliance with a nurse, therapist, clergy, or support group leader, people are often encouraged to "pay it forward" to help themselves and subsequently help others in the aftermath of trauma. We also recognize that all of the women in any of the four studies discussed in this book had a span of at least five years that distanced them from the trauma event. For many women, the timeline was well beyond five years. This, in turn, gave them time to process their experience and have some healing. An added advantage was the realization of support from family, friends, and colleagues. None of the women mentioned in this book were alone without support. We suggest that the aforementioned explanations may give credence to the fact that all participants experienced some degree of PTG as represented by the five domains outlined in the PTG conceptual model.

As nurses, researchers, authors, and professors, we are immensely grateful to the women who participated in the four research studies explored in this book. They shared their stories of trauma with us to capture their experiences in a research context and to help other women who are dealing with adversity. Their narratives touched our hearts, minds, and souls as nurses. The stories were sad, painful, gut-wrenching, candid, and meaningful. The women were courageous to share their stories of trauma, loss, and devastation with us. Their words sought to inform, empower, and comfort others in their time of need. Their efforts to offer anticipatory guidance by telling their stories were thoughtful, generous, and brave. As healthcare professionals, we savored the sharing that occurred as the women told their stories. They mentioned coping, grieving, seeking support, finding meaning, and rediscovering themselves. They spoke of caring, compassion, empathy, and working to help others.

After transcribing audio-recorded interviews and listening to the women's voices repeatedly, we believe that we gained significant insight into their traumas. There was sorrow and devastation with loss, fear and terror with the realization of one's possible demise, a deep hurt accompanying one's diminished self-esteem, and an ultimate sense of betrayal with intimate partner abuse. We acquired a valuable understanding of the totality of the traumatic experience as well as the uphill journey in the direction of PTG. The women's journeys were individual, and there was no specific trajectory to PTG. The women were unique in their traumas as well as in the domains of PTG. Some women gravitated toward new possibilities, while others recognized a basic appreciation for life. The most universal testimony was the acknowledgment of a strong support system to mediate fear, offer comfort, and provide a positive presence.

The women's stories had a much more profound effect on our lives than we anticipated. We gained increased respect and admiration for the strength and fortitude of the women participating in these four research studies. It was astonishingly brave of them to bear their souls to us in a research context exploring negative experiences. Many shared with us the fact that the details of their trauma remained somewhat hidden from family and friends to spare their loved ones the pain they endured. Yet, they were amazingly candid in the interviews with us because of the nature of our research and to help others who may befall similar traumas. We gained increased respect, appreciation, and admiration for our research participants. They were courageous, caring, compassionate, and empathetic.

The voices of women are important for humankind. We are all life-long learners and can benefit from knowledge development about PTG as well as information about PTSD and positive coping behaviors. The purpose of this book was to describe and explore PTG in four distinct groups of women who had previously experienced trauma. We sought to inform our readers of the possibility of PTG in women who had experienced the loss of a spouse or partner, the loss of a child, the frightening scenario of a close brush with death, or the betrayal demonstrated by intimate partner abuse.

When examining the research findings, two distinct elements regarding PTG stand out. First, not every person who has experienced trauma sees facets of PTG in their life. Some people may not move in the direction of PTG for some time, and others may never move in this direction. It is possible to remain stuck in sorrow and pain. Second, there is no specific timeline for PTG. While we generally think of a process as having a beginning, a middle, and an end, PTG may be an open-ended process that ebbs and flows with the dynamics of a person's life. There may not be a finite endpoint.

Each chapter showcased new information about PTG. Chapter 1 presented pertinent information about PTSD. Without this chronology, we would not be able to outline the domains of the PTG framework of Tedeschi and Calhoun (1995, 1996, 2004) and lay the groundwork necessary to study the four groups of women discussed in this book. Chapter 2 introduced the aforementioned PTG model and explained that when humans are faced with adversity, the restoration of psychological functioning and well-being is a possibility. While traumatic events can lead to feelings of distress, extreme sadness, vulnerability, and anger; people can also emerge from adversity and make positive changes in their lives. Chapter 3 is based on our first research study, PTG in women who have lost their spouse or partner to death. The women told their stories of loss and differentiated whether the loss was anticipated or unanticipated. This chapter showcased themes such as social support, empathy, and compassion. Chapter 4 dealt with women who had lost a child to death. In this chapter, two grandmothers joined the group of grieving mothers to tell their stories. Themes described the myriad of emotions encountered by the women. Chapter 5 highlighted the experiences of women who had a close brush with death themselves. Themes recounted their fear, coping, and recovery. Some of these women had out-of-body or near-death experiences encapsulated in their close brush with death. Chapter 6 told the stories of women who had been victims of intimate partner abuse, which entailed emotional or physical abuse, or both. Themes pointed to the acknowledgment of abuse, betrayal, gaslighting, and destruction of self-esteem. Chapter 7 provides a summary of proven therapeutic modalities, self-help initiatives, clinical practice, education, and research recommendations for future research. The current chapter provides our final and concluding thoughts as clinicians, authors, and researchers.

This book offers hope to women who find themselves in adverse circumstances. The stories contained in the book via a research context capture the trials and tribulations, but also the triumphs and victories, of the women who shared their narratives with us. Their voices are represented in excerpts from verbatim transcriptions taken from in-depth personal interviews. All names were changed for privacy and confidentiality, but their words remain true. The book is replete with vivid descriptions, soulful comments, and intricate details regarding the women's lives and the impact of the traumatic event. Their stories speak of actions, behaviors, observations, and precious words that will never be forgotten. These past experiences informed and shaped the future of the research participants.

It is paramount to remember that people suffering from PTSD are continually reminded of the original traumatic event, and their thoughts and feelings associated with the event are reexperienced in vivid dreams and flashbacks. Historical accounts tell us that those who suffered from childhood abuse or rape, those who lived in New York City when the twin towers fell on September 11, 2001, and those who were injured in a serious accident or natural disaster often have feelings of helplessness or despair. Many find themselves emotionally numb, prone to insomnia and other sleep difficulties, misusing alcohol, abusing drugs, and in some cases contemplating suicide. It is a well-known fact that the suicide rate for veterans of the wars in Iraq and Afghanistan is alarmingly high in the United States.

The personal stresses discussed in this book relate to major life events, but in studying the phenomenon of PTG, we must acknowledge that other events may cause significant life disruptions that also take their toll on a person's well-being. Some of these may be the loss of employment, divorce or separation, mental illness, failure in college, poverty, being a victim of crime, and a host of other serious disappointments and setbacks. In addition, some effects of personal stress may be lingering. For example, being a victim of rape or violence, being disfigured from burns, not being able to find gainful employment, or having your home in foreclosure are all difficult and painful circumstances. These occurrences may cause a person to suffer consequences long after the actual event.

People habitually use coping mechanisms to help manage the stress in their lives. They may not even be aware that they are doing this. These mechanisms serve a protective function to control, reduce, or learn to tolerate the threats or triggers that generate stress. In most stressful situations, people use both emotion-focused and problem-focused modalities and strategies to maintain some sort of equilibrium. An emotion-focused strategy might be to accept sympathy, allow someone to help, or by making a concerted effort to be positive. Problem-focused coping tries to change or alter the issue that is responsible for stress. It may involve a behavior change or the formulation of an action plan to combat stress.

We believe that it is time for a paradigm shift with a greater focus on PTG, especially when PTSD is recognized and treated with whatever therapeutic modalities are most effective for the person. There can be light at the end of the tunnel for those who have difficulty functioning after trauma. Their well-being can return even though their life has changed because of trauma.

We are not minimizing PTSD, but we are emphasizing the possibility of PTG. Healthcare providers need to embrace a positive trajectory for patients, families, and themselves. Wellness needs to be embedded in the fabric of human beings both personally and professionally. The concept of PTG needs to be introduced in educational programs for those entering the healthcare field. It should begin in academic institutions and continue into clinical practice for nurses, physicians, and other healthcare workers. It is universally recognized that humans have an innate possibility for growth if they receive education about PTG and choose to explore PTG rather than focus solely on PTSD.

Dealing with trauma can teach a person a lot about themselves. It can serve as a wake-up call to put things in perspective. It can spark questions and cause people to revisit their priorities. It can be a powerful reminder of what truly matters in life. A traumatic event may cause some to realize that they want to spend more time with loved ones rather than work long hours for financial gain. Some may decide to make amends with estranged family members or friends, especially if the separation was the result of a trivial disagreement. Others may discover they want to work less and pursue enjoyable activities. Things once considered important, such as a premier residence or driving an expensive car, may descend on the priority list. Following one's passions may take precedence over living up to the expectations of others and society. Surviving trauma may lead to the conclusion that life is short and that you will not know when your last day will come or if you will have a last day with someone you love.

Most people search for connection with others, meaning in life, and love. They want to be seen, heard, understood, and appreciated. They want their life to count. Magical moments with family, friends, and co-workers should not be overlooked or forgotten. After a close brush with death, the loss of a loved one, or intimate partner abuse, people want to have hope for the future. They want life to get better and do not want to give up on life.

In summary, we are tremendously grateful to the brave women who came forward and identified themselves to us for participation in our research endeavor. Each woman had a highly individual experience with a unique set of psychological and social variables. Each voice needed to be heard, understood, validated, and comforted. We acknowledge that there is no specific roadmap outlining the path to PTG. Barriers or obstacles to PTG can be acute, chronic, and of varying degrees. Time is framed by a variety of individual, contextual, and cultural features. Life after trauma is a very personal journey filled with positives and negatives, ups and downs, and starts and stops. A "new normal" begins with a change in a person's life.

## References

Tedeschi, R., & Calhoun, L. (1995). *Trauma and transformation: Growth in the aftermath of suffering*. Sage.

Tedeschi, R., & Calhoun, L. (1996). The posttraumatic growth inventory: Measuring the positive legacy of trauma. *Journal of Traumatic Stress, 9*(3), 455–472.

Tedeschi, R., & Calhoun, L. (2004). Posttraumatic growth: Conceptual foundations and empirical evidence. *Psychological Inquiry, 15*(1), 1–18.

# AFTERWORD

My memory is vivid of the day I received a call from a friend, colleague, and mentor, Dr. Beth Scannell-Desch, regarding the research she and her twin sister, Dr. Mary Ellen Doherty, were about to conduct. She shared that the focus of the study was on posttraumatic growth (PTG). I was transfixed and intrigued by the possibilities and immediately wanted to know about the study design, method, participants, and interview guide that would explore this phenomenon of human growth after trauma and loss. This research was not only exciting but significant and timely.

For the writing of this book, Scannell-Desch & Doherty conducted and compiled four qualitative studies. Each study focused on a distinct group of women that individually and collectively have experienced spousal loss, child loss, a close brush with death, and domestic abuse. Rich descriptions and themes coalesced, and what resounded were the voices of these courageous women proclaiming, "We are here. We are still standing. We are stronger." In reading each of the studies, an emerging pattern of hope triumphantly arises from each page. In each narrative, we walk with these women as they share their tragic lived experiences and what Tedeschi and Calhoun (1996) described as the positive legacy of trauma (Tedeschi et al., 2018). This book is a moving tribute to these women.

The research then unfolds to move beyond the simple identification and definition of the posttraumatic growth phenomenon into the journey of each participant's experience and how they moved from a place of the inherent resilience of merely bouncing back to life after trauma into the reality of personal transformation. This research provides a greater understanding of human becoming when encountering great adversity and challenge.

These nurse scholars share the findings of their research studies synthesizing and extracting new knowledge on posttraumatic growth and research-supported interventions to inform both trauma survivors who read this book and the professionals who care for them. It reassures the reader that no one is alone and that hope prevails. Through primary, secondary, or vicarious trauma, women may experience adversity and suffer at some point in their lives, and nurses are well-situated to provide therapeutic support and guidance to others as they navigate the experience of trauma.

The authors posit that care needs to be tailored to each woman, their unique circumstances, and where they may be in their nonlinear post-trauma-growth trajectory. PTG has no timeline but occurs in an individual's own time, and there may be no guarantee that they will even experience it. If one does experience growth after trauma, there is a moving beyond to a higher level of functioning, a greater appreciation of life, enhanced personal strength, deeper relationships with others, and an openness to the possibilities in life.

Humanistic psychologist Abraham Maslow (1969) introduced the concept of self-actualization as the final stage of his theory on the hierarchy of needs. Maslow viewed self-actualization as a rite of passage that allows the individual to go beyond the single self into self-transcendence. He believed that it is possible to grow from adversity, often integrating painful wounds of the past that have disrupted one's worldview, causing chaos and confusion. Posttraumatic growth requires orienting to inherent strengths, acknowledging and attending to residual pain, and taking charge of the narrative that defines one's life.

This book is thought-provoking and inspiring. It is both significant and timely. It is significant in that it specifically addresses a gap in the abuse literature focusing on posttraumatic growth in women survivors of domestic violence in the United States. It is timely in that traumatic events are becoming commonplace in our nation and posttraumatic stress statistics are on the rise. I applaud the authors for turning a scientific gaze upon this most important phenomenon. Well done.

**Colleen Fleming-Damon, Ph.D., ANP-BC, ACHPN, FT, CNE**
**Hospice and Palliative Nurse Practitioner-Thanatologist**

### References

Maslow, A. H. (1969). The farther reaches of human nature. *Journal of Transpersonal Psychology*, *1*(1), 1–9.

Tedeschi, R. G., Shakespeare-Finch, J., Taku, K., & Calhoun, L. G. (2018). *Posttraumatic growth: Theory, research, and applications*. Routledge.

Tedeschi, R., & Calhoun, L. (1996). The posttraumatic growth inventory: Measuring the positive legacy of trauma. *Journal of Traumatic Stress*, *9*(3), 455–472.

# GLOSSARY

**Attention deficit disorder (ADD)**   A behavioral condition usually diagnosed during childhood. It is characterized by symptoms including inattention, hyperactivity, and impulsivity.

**Bacterial spinal meningitis**   A bacterial infection of the membranes (meninges) surrounding the brain and spinal cord.

**Beck Depression Inventory (BDI)**   This is widely used to screen for depression and to measure behavioral manifestations and severity of depression. The BDI can be used for ages 13 to 80. The inventory contains 21 self-report items, which individuals complete using multiple-choice response formats.

**Bilirubin**   A red-orange compound that occurs in the normal catabolic pathway that breaks down heme in vertebrates. This catabolism is a necessary process in the body's clearance of waste products that arise from the destruction of aged or abnormal red blood cells. High bilirubin levels, or hyperbilirubinemia, means an excessive accumulation of bilirubin in the blood.

**Bleb**   A bleb is an air-filled cyst that forms on the lung pleura. Most are asymptomatic but also can cause a lung to collapse.

**Cardiac tamponade**   Compression of the heart due to fluid buildup in the sac surrounding the heart.

**CellCept**   CellCept (Mycophenolate mofetil) is used to prevent organ rejection in people at least 3 months old who have received a liver, kidney, or heart transplant. Mycophenolate mofetil is also used with other medicines to prevent organ transplant rejection.

**Clostridium deficile**   A bacteria that causes serious diarrheal infection of the large intestine. Can lead to severe dehydration and can be life-threatening if not treated.

**Cognitive behavioral therapy (CBT)**   This is a psychosocial intervention that aims to reduce symptoms of various mental health conditions, primarily depression and anxiety disorders Cognitive behavioral therapy is one of the most effective means of treatment for substance abuse and co-occurring mental health disorders. CBT is a common form of talk therapy based on the combination of the basic principles from behavioral and cognitive psychology.

**Cognitive processing therapy (CPT)**   Cognitive processing therapy (CPT) is a type of cognitive behavioral therapy that helps people with PTSD change their unhelpful beliefs related to the trauma. It is a short-term, evidence-based psychotherapy that can be delivered in individual or group sessions. It is a recommended first-line treatment for service members, veterans, and survivors of traumatic experiences with PTSD.

**Complicated grief**   People with this condition are caught up in rumination about the circumstances of the death, worry about its consequences, or excessive avoidance of reminders of the loss.

**Conceptual frameworks**   Used in research studies to provide a focus. Describe a perspective in which key factors or elements such as constructs or variables link to relationships. Conceptual frameworks set boundaries and provide a foundation for the construction of a research study.

**Covid-19**   A pandemic caused by a virus that spread worldwide in 2019–2021, causing many deaths. Coronaviruses are a family of viruses that can cause illnesses such as the common cold, severe acute respiratory syndrome (SARS), and Middle East respiratory syndrome (MERS). In 2019, a new coronavirus was identified as the cause of a disease outbreak that originated in China.

**Crohn's disease**   Crohn's disease is an inflammatory bowel disease that causes chronic inflammation of the gastrointestinal tract, which usually results in chronic diarrhea that may be bloody. There is no cure for this disease, but it can be managed with medications, diet, and stress reduction measures.

**DiGeorge syndrome**   A disorder caused when a small part of chromosome 22 is missing. This deletion results in the poor development of several body systems. Medical problems commonly associated with this syndrome include heart defects, poor immune system function, a cleft palate, complications related to low levels of calcium in the blood, and delayed development with behavioral and emotional problems.

**Dilation and curettage (D&C)**   A procedure to remove tissue from inside the uterus. Healthcare providers perform dilation and curettage to diagnose and treat certain uterine conditions, such as heavy bleeding, or to clear the uterine lining after a miscarriage, retained placental parts, or abortion.

**Emergency medical technician (EMT)**   A specially trained medical technician certified to provide basic emergency services including CPR before and during transportation to a hospital.

**Eye movement desensitization and reprocessing (EMDR)**   A mental health treatment technique involving moving your eyes a specific way while you process traumatic memories. EMDR's goal is to help you heal from trauma or other distressing life experiences.

**Gaslighting**   The practice of psychologically manipulating someone into questioning their sanity, memory, or powers of reasoning.

**Gastric volvulus**   An abnormal rotation of all or part of the stomach around one of its axes. It is a diagnostic emergency and causes an acute bowel obstruction.

**Guillain–Barre syndrome**   Guillain-Barre syndrome is an auto-immune disorder where antibodies are directed against the peripheral nerves. Symptoms may include tingling sensations in the peripheries, which may worsen leading to paralysis.

**Hepatic necrosis**   An extensive and rapid death of parenchymal cells in the liver, often due to exposure to toxic materials. Can result from hyperbilirubinemia that is not treated.

**Hyperbilirubinemia**   This means you have an excessive accumulation of bilirubin. A build-up of excess bilirubin causes jaundice—a condition that causes the skin, mucous membranes, and white part of the eyes to take on a yellow hue. High bilirubin is common in newborns because their liver is still learning how to efficiently clear bilirubin.

**Hypoplastic left heart**   Occurs when parts of the left side of the heart (mitral valve, left ventricle, aortic valve, and aorta) do not develop completely. The condition is present at birth (congenital).

**Immunoglobulins IgG**   IgG is the most common type of antibody in your blood and other body fluids. These antibodies protect you against infection by remembering which germs you've been exposed to before. If those germs come back, your immune system knows to attack them.

**Impact Event Scale–Revised (IES-R)**   A 22-item self-report measure that assesses subjective distress caused by traumatic events. The IES-R contains seven additional items related to the hyperarousal symptoms of PTSD, which were not included in the original IES. Respondents are asked to identify a specific stressful life event and then indicate how much they were distressed or bothered during the past seven days by each difficulty listed.

**Institutional Review Board (IRB)**   Refers to a group whose function is to review research to assure the protection of the rights and welfare of human subjects. Sometimes called the Ethics Committee.

**Lyme disease**   An illness caused by borrelia bacteria. Humans usually get Lyme disease from the bite of a tick carrying the bacteria. Ticks that can carry borrelia bacteria live throughout most of the United States. But Lyme disease is most common in the upper Midwest and the northeastern and mid-Atlantic states. It's also common in Europe and south-central and southeastern Canada.

**Methicillin-resistant *Staphylococcus aureus* (MRSA)**   A staph infection that is difficult to treat because of resistance to some antibiotics. Staph infections—including those caused by MRSA—can spread in hospitals, other healthcare facilities, and in the community where you live, work, and go to school.

**Mindfulness-Based Stress Reduction Program (MBSR)**   A meditation therapy, though originally designed for stress management, it is being used for treating a variety of illnesses such as depression, anxiety, chronic pain, cancer, diabetes mellitus, hypertension, and auto-immune disorders.

**Myeloproliferative essential thrombocytosis neoplasia**   A chronic myeloproliferative neoplasm (MPN) characterized by an increased number of platelets in the blood. It is most commonly diagnosed in women over 50 years of age. Complications frequently involve blood clotting and bleeding.

**Myocardial infarction (MI)**   A heart attack. It occurs when blood flow decreases or stops in the coronary artery of the heart, causing damage to the heart muscle.

**Near-death experience (NDE)**   The conscious, semiconscious, or recollected experience of someone who is approaching or has temporarily begun the process of dying, for example, during a cardiac arrest that is followed by resuscitation.

**Near-Death Experience Scale**   A scale to measure NDEs. The NDE Scale asks 16 questions about the NDE content and is the most validated scale to help distinguish NDEs from other types of experiences. For an experience to be classified as an NDE, there has to be a score of seven or above on the NDE Scale.

**Neonatal Intensive Care Unit (NICU)**   Specialized intensive care unit that cares for newborns shortly after birth because of conditions requiring special monitoring and intensive care. Some of the medical conditions can include prematurity, low birth weight, respiratory distress, cardiac irregularities, birth defects, and other serious conditions.

**Omentum**   A sheet of fat or tissue that is covered by the peritoneum and surrounds or supports the organs and intestines in the abdomen. It has two parts: the greater omentum, which hangs down from the stomach, and the lesser omentum, which connects the stomach to the liver.

**Pneumothorax**   A condition in which air accumulates in the pleural space, causing it to expand and thus compress the underlying lung, which may then collapse. The pleural space is a cavity formed by the two pleural membranes that line the thoracic cavity and cover the lungs. Symptoms include sudden onset of sharp, one-sided chest pain and shortness of breath.

**Polyhydramnios**   Excessive accumulation of amniotic fluid, which is the fluid that surrounds the baby in the uterus during pregnancy. Polyhydramnios occurs in about 1 to 2 percent of pregnancies. Most cases of polyhydramnios are mild and result from a gradual buildup of amniotic fluid during the second half of pregnancy. Severe polyhydramnios may cause shortness of breath, preterm labor, or other signs and symptoms of distress.

**Posttraumatic growth (PTG)**   The positive personal transformations that can occur in the aftermath of trauma. Positive psychological changes occur after a struggle from traumatic, painful, and highly challenging life circumstances.

**Posttraumatic Growth Inventory (PTGI)**   A quantitative 21-item scale used by researchers to measure PTG.

**Posttraumatic Growth Model**   Doctors Tedeschi and Calhoun at the University of North Carolina–Charlotte identified five domains of posttraumatic growth: (1) a greater appreciation of life, (2) improved relationships with others, (3) increased personal strength, (4) openness to new possibilities, and (5) spiritual growth.

**Posttraumatic Stress Checklist (PCL-5)**   The PCL-5 is a 20-item questionnaire, corresponding to the DSM-5 symptom criteria for PTSD. The wording of PCL-5 items reflects both changes to existing symptoms and the addition of new symptoms in DSM-5. The self-report rating scale is 0–4 for each symptom, reflecting a change from 1 to 5 in the DSM-IV version.

**Post-traumatic stress disorder (PTSD)**   A mental and behavioral disorder that can develop because of exposure to a traumatic event, such as sexual assault, warfare, tornados, aircraft or automobile crashes, earthquakes, fires, domestic violence, or other threats to a person's life. Symptoms may include disturbing thoughts, feelings, or dreams related to the events; mental or physical distress to trauma-related cues; attempts to avoid trauma-related cues, alterations in the way a person thinks and feels, and an increase in the fight-or-flight response. These symptoms last for more than a month after the event.

**Prednisone**  A corticosteroid medicine used to decrease inflammation and keep your immune system in check, if it is overactive. Prednisone is used to treat allergic disorders, skin conditions, ulcerative colitis, Crohn's disease, arthritis, lupus, psoriasis, asthma, chronic obstructive pulmonary disease (COPD), and many more conditions.

**Prolonged exposure therapy (PET)**  A form of behavior therapy and cognitive behavioral therapy designed to treat post-traumatic stress disorder (PTSD). It is characterized by two main treatment procedures—imaginal and in vivo exposures. Imaginal exposure is repeated "on-purpose" retelling of the trauma memory. In vivo exposure involves confronting situations that are avoided because they are associated with the trauma.

**Propofol**  Marketed as Diprivan, a short-acting medication that results in a decreased level of consciousness and a lack of memory for events. Its uses include the induction and maintenance of general anesthesia, sedation for mechanically ventilated adults, and procedural sedation.

**Purposive sampling technique**  Purposive sampling is a nonprobability sampling technique used in research to select individuals or groups of individuals that meet specific criteria relevant to the research question or objective. It is also known as subjective sampling.

**Qualitative content analysis**  A type of qualitative research tool or method that focuses on analyzing content in various mediums, the most common of which is written words in documents. In qualitative research, it is a common procedure to analyze data from interviews and focus group verbatim transcriptions.

**Respiratory syncytial virus (RSV)**  Causes infections of the lungs and respiratory tract. It is so common that most children have been infected with the virus by age 2. This virus can also infect adults.

**Selective serotonin reuptake inhibitors (SSRIs)**  Selective serotonin reuptake inhibitors (SSRIs) are the most commonly prescribed antidepressants. They can ease symptoms of moderate to severe depression, are relatively safe, and typically cause fewer side effects than other types of antidepressants do.

**Septic shock**  A serious medical condition that can occur when an infection in your body causes extremely low blood pressure and organ failure due to sepsis. Septic shock is life-threatening and requires immediate medical treatment.

**Snowball sampling technique**  Snowball sampling is a nonprobability sampling method or a technique whereby currently enrolled research participants help recruit future subjects for a study.

**Stepford Wives**  A 1975 film in which a family of four moves from New York City to the Connecticut community of Stepford, where the wife comes to find the women live unwaveringly subservient lives to their husbands.

**Subdural hematoma**  A type of bleeding in which a collection of blood gathers between the inner layer of the dura mater and the arachnoid mater of the meninges surrounding the brain. It usually results from tears in bridging veins that cross the subdural space. Usually results from a fall or blow to the head.

**Total parenteral nutrition (TPN)**  A way of supplying all the nutritional needs of the body by bypassing the digestive system and dripping nutrient solution directly into a vein. The goal of the treatment is to correct or prevent malnutrition. The method is used when someone can't or shouldn't receive feedings or fluids by mouth.

**Toxic megacolon**   An acute form of colonic distension characterized by a very dilated colon (megacolon), accompanied by abdominal distension (bloating), and sometimes fever, abdominal pain, or shock.

**Tracheostomy**   A tracheostomy, also known as a tracheotomy, is a small surgical opening that is made through the front of the neck into the windpipe, or trachea. A curved plastic tube, known as a tracheostomy tube, is placed through the hole, allowing air to flow in and out of the windpipe. The tube does not extend into the lungs.

**Transesophageal endoscopy (TEE)**   A TEE is different than other forms of echocardiogram or ultrasounds because it takes pictures from within your body rather than outside of it. Your provider uses an endoscope to carefully guide a small transducer down your throat and esophagus. The transducer is a device that makes sound waves.

**VACTERL**   Stands for vertebral defects, anal atresia, cardiac defects, trachea-esophageal fistula, renal abnormalities, and limb abnormalities. Most VACTERL babies have at least three of these defects.

**Zeljam**   An oral prescription medication approved to treat moderately to severely active rheumatoid arthritis, psoriatic arthritis, and ulcerative colitis. It also comes in an extended-release formulation, Xeljanz XR. Both formulations contain the active ingredient tofacitinib.

**Z-plasty**   A surgical procedure performed on burn patients that have lower facial burns affecting the chin and neck to free up tissue so that the chin is not pulled down toward the chest.

# INDEX

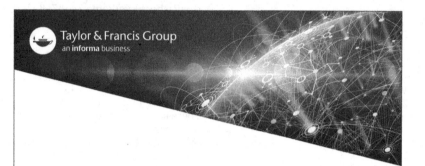

Taylor & Francis Group
an **informa** business

# Taylor & Francis eBooks

## www.taylorfrancis.com

A single destination for eBooks from Taylor & Francis
with increased functionality and an improved user
experience to meet the needs of our customers.

90,000+ eBooks of award-winning academic content in
Humanities, Social Science, Science, Technology, Engineering,
and Medical written by a global network of editors and authors.

### TAYLOR & FRANCIS EBOOKS OFFERS:

A streamlined
experience for
our library
customers

A single point
of discovery
for all of our
eBook content

Improved
search and
discovery of
content at both
book and
chapter level

## REQUEST A FREE TRIAL
### support@taylorfrancis.com

 Routledge
Taylor & Francis Group

 CRC Press
Taylor & Francis Group